EVERYTHING YOU ALWAYS WANTED TO KNOW ABOUT

POTASSIUM

BUT WERE TOO TIRED

TO ASK

How Potassium Affects
- *high blood pressure*
- *fatigue*
- *the aging process*
- *alcoholism*
- *headaches*
  and more. . .

by Betty Kamen, Ph.D.

Potassium-sodium graphics by Paul Kamen

Nutrition Encounter, Inc., Novato, California

All of the facts in this book have been very carefully researched and have been drawn from the scientific literature. In no way, however, are any of the suggestions meant to take the place of advice given by physicians. Please consult a medical or health professional should the need for one be indicated.

Nutrition Encounter, Inc., 1992
Box 2736
Novato, CA 94948

Printed in the United States of America
First Printing: 1992
Second Printing: 1992
ISBN 0-944501-06-0

Dedicated to:

Larry Jordan

whose unusual perspicacity
has opened many doors for many people.

CONTENTS

Conditions discussed in Part II

OTHER BOOKS BY BETTY KAMEN, PH.D.

Betty Kamen is an award-winning journalist and photojournalist, with graduate degrees in psychology and nutrition education. She is an internationally-known lecturer, radio/TV host, and the author of many major books, hundreds of articles, and several tapes on various aspects of health and nutrition. For many years, she hosted *Nutrition 57* on WMCA in New York, followed by *Nutrition Watch* on KNBR in San Francisco.

ACKNOWLEDGMENTS

Paul Kamen,
       for the potassium cell-membrane
       schematics and food charts

Si Kamen,
       for support and commitment

Margie Kern,
       for herbal knowledge

Perle Kinney,
       for being there

Graphic Arts:
       New Vision Technologies, Inc.
       TechPool Studios
       ProArt Multi Ad Services
       T/Maker Company

FOREWORD

Betty Kamen is gradually becoming an updated and improved version of Betty Crocker. Yes, she is a symbol of the *joy of good food*; but more, she is a teacher, able to translate nutrition science into helpful ideas for everyone interested in optimal health. In this latest book, Dr. Kamen shows us how to understand and obtain adequate potassium in our food. That she has written on this neglected subject at all is admirable, for potassium deficiency is the hidden side of chronic fatigue, high blood pressure, headache and, in fact, is an important contributor to all forms of degenerative disease. Betty opens our eyes to this vital knowledge, guiding us quickly from the medical findings to the dietary applications.

You will be healthier, enjoy more energy and well-being, and ward off aging and illness better after you read Betty Kamen's new book. Remember, potassium is not found in vitamin pills, and it is not easily available or cheap by medical prescription. But it is plentiful in everyday foods if you know which to choose. Betty tells you why potassium is so important and shows you how to get it naturally in healthful, good-tasting foods.

For those who find it difficult to adjust their lifestyles, suggestions for safe and practical potassium supplementation are included.

Richard A. Kunin, M.D.
San Francisco, CA
Medical Nutrition and Health Medicine
Past-president, Orthomolecular Medical Society
Author, *MegaNutrition*

AUTHOR'S NOTES

While groping for the best possible title for this book, a friend suggested, "Potassium or Die." Not bad. It was dramatic, to the point, and it spoke the truth. Well, close to the truth. Of course no one could live without potassium. Potassium, along with sodium, is the most biologically important of the alkaline minerals. The emphasis here is that too many people are nutritionally potassium-deficient. Consequently, they lack life's luster; they suffer various and sundry disorders; they may wilt when they could bloom. *Perhaps that is a kind of death.*

Had this book been written a decade or two earlier, its contents would have been somewhat different. No doubt the underlying messages would have been the same, but our full comprehension would have been far less clear and proof of the concepts developed far less convincing. Terms like "gut feeling" or "theory" or "just a hypothesis" would weave through the chapters. High technology of current vintage enables us to define the very detailed information with more accuracy. And as this is happening, the larger and broader view is becoming better focused.

Recently, as a guest at a small conference of physicians, my attention was piqued when one of the doctors, Peter H. C. Mutke, M.D., a general practitioner in the Pleasant Hill and Walnut Creek areas of northern California, shared the fact that a large percentage of his patients who had chronic fatigue syndrome claimed to feel much better on a liquid product containing potassium and herbs. A lively discussion ensued among the physicians: What was responsible for the reduction in worn-down feelings? Was it the potassium in the elixir? The herbs? Both? Another physician, Richard A. Kunin, M.D., of San Francisco, related his success with potassium supplementation and headaches.

Inspired by these challenges and by a new awareness imparted to me, which came from many long conversations with my friend Larry Jordan (to whom this book is dedicated), I set out to find some answers. What started as a "booklet" project expanded as I learned more and more about the interactions of sodium and potassium — in particular, the impact these have on how you feel, how you age, how much energy you have, and even on serious disease states.

My groundwork revealed a few biological facts for which the word *awesome* is an understatement:

> *As often as a thousand times a second, sodium ions and potassium ions exchange places to inform your brain about size, distance, patterns, color.*

> *As long as life continues, potassium helps to govern its processes.*

> *A trail of electricity, caused by sodium-potassium maneuvers, flashes so rapidly across your heart that all its cells appear to beat as one.*

> *Malaise and fatigue, are the most common deficiency symptoms when potassium deficits are chronic.*

And that was only the beginning!

Betty Kamen

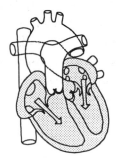

HEART
ACTION
(dependent on potassium)

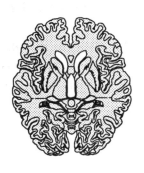

BRAIN
FUNCTION

(dependent on potassium)

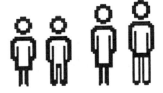

LIFE
PROCESSES
(dependent on potassium)

LACK OF ENERGY

(may be symptom of
potassium deficiency)

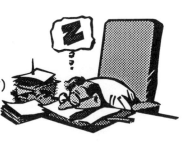

PROLOGUE

PROLOGUE

*in which Diana feels tired,
so tired, dead tired
(a little soap opera)*

DIANA FALLS APART

Diana knew *exactly* what time it was, yet she glanced at the office clock again. The knots in the pit of her stomach, already taut, pulled even closer. Her sitter had informed her about going home early this particular day. Her husband was out of town. Her mother was not available. Mr. Smythe had not yet called with his promise of a yes-or-no response to the critically important proposal she had labored over for weeks. (Her auto mechanic, however, had been in touch several times — with car-repair quotes beyond the limit of her Visa balance.) A rotten day.

Diana's brain cells were battling. Go? Stay? Go!

Just as the "depart" message gained the lead, her call came through. "I have good news," Smythe said. "The Board approved your idea." Diana held back a squeal of delight. Good thing, because Smythe wasn't finished.

"Well, *almost* approved," he continued. "One segment requires more graphics. And we need them by morning."

Guarded excitement. She had the assignment — *almost*. Why couldn't they understand her proposal without elaboration? Three more hours of tough, hard work. Maybe four or five. There was that funny feeling in her head. And she was tired. So tired. Dead tired.

Diana waited impatiently for the elevator. The late-day sun pierced through a window, accenting a harsh vision of herself in a nearby mirror. As she caught sight of her spotlighted reflection, she was startled at the image gazing back at her — and for a brief moment deeply affected by how old she looked. A friend had told her about a "tonic" that supposedly helped age-reversal and helped fatigue. She hadn't paid much attention. She'd call Sally tonight.

Was she going to get one of those awful headaches again? She had a history of similar difficulties — nausea, fatigue, occasional blurry vision, other characteristics of migraine. But no physician had been able to pinpoint the precise problem or suggest a remedy that worked.

As she had advanced in years, Diana's symptoms, although still present, were not as severe. Oh, she still had severe menstrual cramps, but didn't everyone? Why was she feeling *this* ill and looking *this* old? Or was she, perhaps, viewing herself from the midnight side of things because of her uneasy day? Would it all go away? Or was something seriously wrong?

No cab in sight. Diana could see the bus at the depot two blocks away. She *must* make that bus. She ran. Fast. She felt dizzy. Pressured. Hurried. And then it hit: Headache. Heartache. Stop. Rest. Run. Lightheaded. Nausea. Breathless. Strain. Pain. *Diana slumped to the ground.*

Cardiac arrest? Some other underlying cardiac problem? A change in blood pressure? Low blood sugar? A neurological condition? Lung disease? Internal hemorrhage? Simple fainting spell? A nutrient deficiency?

The doctors have some of the answers. Their analyses can determine which part of Diana's's reserves just failed. It is unlikely, however, that more than the usual or obvious will be revealed. The complex network of cellular-level causes won't be unveiled or even discussed and perhaps not even fully understood. Physicians are restrained by uncertainties whose nature hasn't been entirely clarified.

> "There should be a course in medical ignorance so doctors can be aware of what is not yet known."
>
> Lewis Thomas, *The Fragile Species*

The examinations given to Diana will focus on her symptoms. A recent report on diagnostic accuracy, cited in the *Journal of the Royal Academy of Physicians of London*, concludes that medical errors arise for two reasons:

- Clinicians tend to look for single, large and static explanations for clinical events.
- When there are multiple factors involved, errors inherent in each step of the diagnosis are compounded.[1]

 The best that Diana can expect is that the physicians will "shore things up" and offer band-aid remedies.

FUNCTIONAL RESERVE AT THE READY

Many tests are available to help decide the course of treatment. Some of these assessments check your cache of reserves, like exercise stress-tests—examinations which determine your heart's supply of reserve power before a serious illness makes that judgment for you. These audits show that a healthy heart can increase its output six-fold or more. The extra backup enables your heart to shunt more blood to your leg muscles to help you move faster when necessary—to empower you to run to catch a bus two blocks away. At its peak, every organ displays increased capacity ranging from four-to-ten times normal. A multitude of other body systems have extra resources, too. Even specific segments of your salivary glands have reserve cells![2]

Here are a few additional illustrations of organ reserve:

➤Selenium is an antioxidant. When faced with selenium deficiency, a healthy heart has a sufficient reserve of antioxidant-enzyme capacity to cope with oxidative stress.[3]

➤During heart failure, there are novel alterations in cardiac efficiency — virtual life-saving attempts.[4]

➤The safety margin by which your small intestine's capacity to absorb nutrients which exceed requirements is enormously large.[5]

➤Experiments with dogs reveal that when oxygen supplies are reduced, blood flow is maintained in vital organs and the brain, and is redistributed away from the kidneys and liver—protecting your ability to use oxygen efficiently.[7]

➤Bone and skeletal-muscle backup pools provide magnesium when it is deficient in your diet. Thus the liver and other organs appear not to lose magnesium despite the deprivation, demonstrating a selective process in using these reserves.[8]

➤When pancreatic islet tissue is surgically removed from test animals, regrowth occurs — thereby preventing the alteration of glucose tolerance.[9]

➤Kidneys must all but fail before they require outside help. Eighty percent of the nephrons, the functional units of the kidneys, can be destroyed, and waste products will still be adequately excreted.[10]

➤An entire lung and sometimes part of the other one can be removed, and the surgeon could still pronounce the operation successful and the prognosis positive.[11]

➤Sometimes three-quarters of the liver can be eliminated without a life-threatening result. A recent example of organ reserve was demonstrated by the mother who gave part of her liver to her young child. The left lobe of the mother's liver was removed, and most of it was transplanted to the daughter. The mother's liver regenerated the lost tissue within three months.

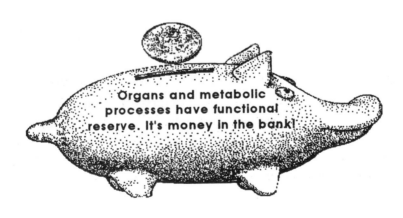

All this surplus function is only used with the occurrence of exceptional demands, anyway — helping to withstand a certain amount of stress. And it helped Diana. *Until today.*

THE DECLINE OF RESERVE

Why were Diana's security assets overdrawn? What had happened to this wonderful, natural gift? The fact is that *the average level of reserve does not remain fixed. Slowly but surely, these resources decline in every living creature!* Like Diana, you are not aware of your waning reserve until you need it and find it is no longer adequate. The reduction of this special protection is present even in animals reared under utopian environments and with super-nutritional diets.

Almighty Time disquiets all things.

Sophocles, two thousand years ago.[12]

So we learn that organ reserve always lessens! The intriguing fact is that *people's reserve powers age at varying rates.*[13] Could the gradual progression that put Diana over the edge have been slowed? Can we learn how to retard the process by examining *causes* — by looking at why different people lose reserve at different rates? I think we can.

Divergence in this slow-down occurs because of:
* individual genetic makeup, determined by heredity
* lifestyle, established by society
* lifestyle, decreed by personal choice
* environment, imposed by local conditions

You can't control it all, but you should be aware that some of your private daily decisions will boost your reserve; others will keep it idling longer than average. How lucky! *You are endowed with the power to make very significant choices.* It wasn't until recently that most of us had the slightest inkling that we could have a say in the matter of our own health. How to make this happen is still ambiguous to many people.

The ebb in functional reserve doesn't necessarily signify illness. It is simply a fact of life, a certainty of each individual's own rate of aging — albeit a different pace in different people. These modifications correlate with disease only when they accelerate beyond the standard, or when they are magnified. As stated in his inimitable style, Lewis Thomas says, "Normal aging is not a disease at all, but a stage of living that cannot be averted or bypassed except in one totally unsatisfactory way."

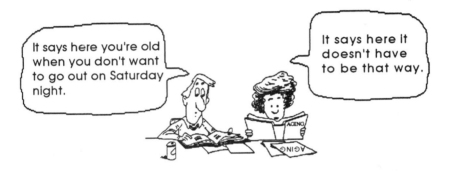

Positive emphasis has been placed on our current older generations' extended years. A report on aging, published in the *American Journal of Clinical Nutrition* (a June 1992 supplement — which arrived in my mail this very day), points out that when we assess a health promotion intervention that has the goal of preventing a disease, a reduction in mortality may not be the best or most sensitive measure of the success or failure of that preventive intervention.

The report also stated that healthy men and women have an important reserve capacity due to good dietary habits (just what has been accented here). But, the researchers caution, the general population has more persons at the *lower* end of the critical health threshold — the time when overall functional reserve no longer satisfies the needs of those individuals.

We also know that each shift in an aging biomarker brings a large number of responses within each person. Examples follow.

➤Reduced water content, a process that occurs gradually with advancing years, affects not only internal organs, but also the tone and elasticity of your skin.

➤Older skin will bruise more easily and heal more slowly.

➤Shrinking of lean body mass is reflected in modifications of skeletal muscle, liver, kidney, spleen, skin, and bone.[14]

➤As the spongy disks between the vertebrae of your spine shrink, you lose height, and, in turn, skin elasticity.

➤Decreased efficiency in nutrient absorption affects *all* metabolic processes.

➤The media has already informed you (more times than you care to hear) about the innumerable and varied consequences of added fat.

And now for two alterations that are of special significance:

➤As your reserve for maintaining electrolyte-balance slackens with aging, the frequency of abnormal circulating concentrations of these minerals increases.[15] (The chief electrolytes include potassium and sodium.)

➤Your kidneys' adaptation to sodium-loading begins its descent in your thirties.[16]

Aging, in any year, touches every part of you. You can't hear it happening — until the aches and pains talk a little louder.

HOW YOUR BODY CHANGES WITH AGE

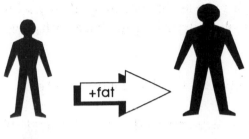

Body fat increases 35%

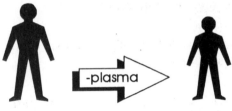

Plasma volume decreases 8%

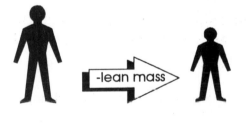

Lean body mass decreases 17%

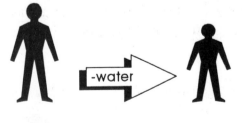

Total body water decreases 17%

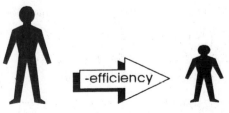

Sodium and potassium efficiency decline significantly

It's the body composition conversions that make you *look* older and *feel* more tired. When Diana caught sight of herself in the mirror, the image took a moment to recognize. She saw the *gestalt*, an overall portrait of an older woman. Her body-composition shifts, although they occurred imperceptibly, were suddenly obvious in the harsh reflection at that stressed moment.

We seldom notice the gradual loss of organ reserve — loss in:
- circulation
- metabolic rate
- hemoglobin
- bone density
- glucose tolerance

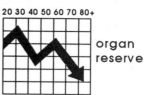

Haven't you noticed differences in family members when you return from a trip, even after a short stay away? You know your son didn't grow a foot in two days. You know your daughter didn't mature over the weekend. Yet they look like they did! And what about yourself? Do you ever see a stranger in a mirror for a fleeting second? Do you perceive your own aging changes in very bright light, perhaps when you adjust your hair in the car mirror on a sunny day? The aging process is a fact of life. *There is, however, a bag of tricks to help slow the pace.*

It isn't easy to give up today's pleasures for tomorrow's benefits. But tomorrow may be the day the rubber band will break, even though stretched no further than yesterday's pull. That's the day you cannot run as fast to catch a bus. No matter what, tomorrow you will be one day older and one day shorter on reserve resources. How much less? *That's an adjustable contract over which you have some influence.*

We admire those who have lived for more than seven or eight decades. They are glorified as outstanding examples of triumph over adversity, but our reverence is tempered by thoughts of old age as a time of decline and dependence; a dwindling of opportunities; a period of despondency. Most of us fear frailty, immobility and intellectual impairment. And we are told that the very old are the fastest growing group in the population!

> The definition of successful aging is the prolongation of minimal illness and disability, coupled with maximum participation in, and enjoyment of, life.

Wouldn't it be wonderful if you could age free of meddling diseases and also imbued with lots of energy? *It's part of the same contract.* Important biological function *can* continue to work superbly for more than one hundred years! You *can* wake to a new morning for the 35,000th time and look forward to a fulfilling day! Yet Diana, like so many others, is having trouble on her 10,000th day! *It doesn't have to be that way!*

As it happens, an accelerated decline in the capacity to retain *mineral* equilibrium plays a major role in responsibility for:
- low energy levels
- many health disorders,
    - life-threatening ones, like heart disease
    - minor daily annoyances, like headaches
- premature aging.

The ratios between two of most important electrolytes — sodium and potassium — and their often-ignored reserve-potential, are of special importance in the context of this book.

AGING SECRETS

AGING SKIN

HOW OLD IS YOUR SKIN?

A New York taxi driver told me he was very astute at judging the age of a woman. All he had to do was look at her elbows. I'm not so sure how accurate the elbow test is, but you can check the age of your own skin with the "Pinch Test," and you can do it when no one is looking!

The pinch test is easy. You don't require a pen or pencil, and you can grade yourself. Place your hand flat on a table, back side up. Pinch a fingerful of loose skin on the back of your hand between your thumb and forefinger of your other hand, and let go. Now note how long it takes until the pinched skin returns to its flat, normal position. The amount of time reveals your skin's relative age.[17]

Women	Men	Skin Age
0 sec	0 sec	10-19
0 sec	0 sec	20-29
1 sec	.5 sec	30-39
3 sec	1 sec	40-49
12 sec	4 sec	50-59
21 sec	20 sec	60-69
1 min	43 sec	over 70

PART 1

*in which we discuss why
sodium-potassium ratios are important
and why they have gone askew.*

UNDERSTANDING
POTASSIUM

THE PROBLEM

Human beings are designed to live in a very special kind of nutritional setting, one that provides more than just an adequate supply of air, water, and mere food energy. For a food supply to support good health, it has to include an incredibe variety and number of different nutrients: carbohydrates, fats, proteins, vitamins, minerals, and even fiber. Some of these substances are important only in minute quantities — but without them, survival isn't possible. Others are necessary in very specific "partner" relationships.

Nutritional science has barely scratched the surface of the vastly complicated mechanisms by which your body uses these various nutrients to help you power yourself in endless ways — to grow, repair, fight off disease, and reproduce.

It may seem like a contradiction, then, that humans live in so many different geographic environments, even here on earth. This suggests versatility rather than a set of rigorous requirements to be met for good health.

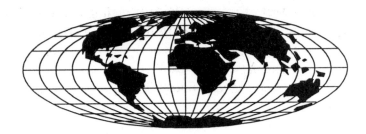

Human cultures have thrived in places that provide completely different sources and mixtures of available nutrients.

However, highly varied natural environments which are conducive to optimal good health have many important aspects in common: *All the food is fresh, unprocessed, unpreserved, and nearly always uncooked.* Pollutants and toxins are usually completely absent or at minimum levels. And minerals occur in specific proportions — ratios that we now know are very different from those in modern diets of the industrialized world.

Despite centuries of progress (and sometimes regression), the scientific understanding of nutrition is still far from complete. And so we are often required to fall back on a philosophical premise: *The food environments of successful preindustrial societies are the ones for which your body has been designed.* A fresh, natural, unprocessed, unpreserved, and mostly uncooked diet describes what our species has been eating for thousands of years — a diet that fills needs not consciously recognized.

In past millennia, food was also plentiful. Anthropologists tell us that for most of human history, fewer than twenty hours a week were devoted to finding food and providing clothing and shelter.

These are efforts we now call "work". There were hard times as well, periods during which food shortages or disease decimated human populations. And of course there have been regions of the world with particularly austere environments where life has always been (and still is) more demanding. But for the most part, humans have lived in relative leisure, eating abundant food, spending the majority of time doing uniquely human things — like telling stories, singing songs, and painting on cave walls. The food environment was hardly ever an issue — and there were no 7-11's, supermarkets or vending machines offering countless processed alternatives.

Like it or not, late twentieth-century humans are built according to those same earlier needs, but in the last five or six decades the character of our food has changed drastically.

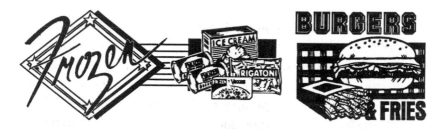

Although we have requirements identical to those of our predecessors, we are exposed to a very different mix of nutrients.

As nutritional research has progressed over time, we have come to understand more and more about these nutrients. Technology has revealed important information about how nutrients relate to each other. Ancient seas were only about one-third as salty as they are today, but they contained a significant amount of potassium, chlorine, calcium, magnesium, and other elements. It is interesting to note that the level of salinity and its ratio to other minerals in these long-ago oceans was more or less the same as that now found in the intercellular fluid and blood of all animals with circulatory systems. This saline level is your genetic heritage.[1]

We also know that sodium, along with potassium, plays a very fundamental role in cell metabolism. These two minerals have extraordinary responsibilities. They are vital to the mechanisms that "power" virtually every living cell in your very human body.

Sodium and potassium control:
- the salinity of the fluid inside and outside your cells
- the acidity or alkalinity of your body
- the entry and exit of many substances wending their way through all body parts enclosed in your skin — substances which help you wave your hand "hello," take deeper breaths when you exercise, enjoy dining out with friends, and to think about your great aunt.

With such important duties, nature must have provided a way for you to secure and utilize the right amount of these elements. And indeed it has! Potassium, the surprising chairperson of the board, is found in abundance in uncooked fruits and vegetables — especially in rinds, husks and stalks of edible plants. Potassium intake has always been very substantial. Sodium, on the other hand, is relatively scarce in natural foods. The original hunter-gatherer humans ingested a diet high in potassium, but low in sodium.[2] Perhaps that's the reason your kidneys easily remove excess potassium from your blood.[3] Your metabolism is more frugal with sodium, simply because under natural conditions there is less of it to be found and eaten. So your body handles sodium with a more sparing kind of metabolism. *Your kidneys actually hoard sodium.*

Average kidneys slow the loss of sodium to a mere 10 milligrams a day if the mineral is in short supply. Daily minimum potassium loss can be as high as 240 milligrams, or 24 times the amount of sodium that is easily excreted![4]

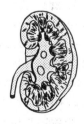

About a decade ago, a report in the *Journal of General Physiology* demonstrated what happens when test animals are deprived of sodium and, in turn, of potassium. The sodium-deficient animals drank more sodium-containing solutions than animals whose diets were amply supplied with sodium. *This adaptation to sodium requirement does not appear to apply to any other nutrient.* Notably, no such differences were observed when solutions of potassium were used on the potassium-deficient animals.[5]

The implication is once again that we are capable of handling far more variations in potassium than in sodium. But (as will be explained in detail later) the relationship between these two substances in your diet is critical for optimal health. While the ideal quantities for potassium and sodium may appear to be neither very large nor significant, the consequences are serious if either level falls below or above the numbers required for good health. The process of conserving sodium is similar in life forms which are as diverse as reptiles, birds, and mammals.

> Grazing animals like deer and cattle seek out salt blocks to balance potassium and sodium intake. These animals consume natural foods, high in potassium and low in sodium — unlike foods in our diet.

However, it cannot be overemphasized that the *ratio* of sodium to potassium is more significant than the absolute amount of either element. The outcome of the relative proportions of these two minerals is somewhat like searching for pistachio nuts in a bowl to which you are also returning the empty shells. As you consume the nuts, it is obvious that the number of "empties" increases while the number of nut-filled shells decreases. Surely you've experienced the advancing difficulty of finding the succulent morsels of nutmeat as this ratio changes. It isn't the *quantity* of nuts remaining in the bowl, but rather the *ratio of nuts to shells* which creates the problem.

And so it is with the ratio of potassium to sodium — the relative quantity of one to the other is the critical factor. The effect intensifies as the ratio moves away from that which your genetic heritage has deemed safe and efficient.

(See chart on facing page. Note the levels of these nutrients found in several intact foods and compare them with those found in processed and cooked versions of today's North American diet — perhaps the very food you have eaten today.)

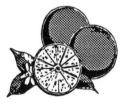

Intact

"Intact" refers to foods which remain unaltered or undis- turbed. Oranges are intact. Orange juice is not, even though manufacturers erro- neously designate both as "natural."

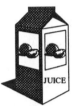

Not Intact

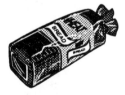

Whole grain bread is more intact than white bread, but is still not an intact food

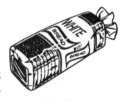

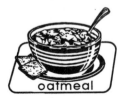
oatmeal

Cookies are not intact. Most whole grain cereals are intact.

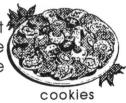

cookies

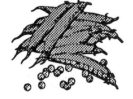

Peas are intact. Pizza is not.

POTASSIUM & SODIUM CONTENT
OF INTACT & DISTURBED FOODS
in milligrams/100 grams food
(100 grams is approximately 3 ½ oz,
or the amount of food equal to the size of a closed fist)

	Potassium	Sodium
Flour, whole	360	3
White bread	100	540
Pork, uncooked	270	65
Bacon, uncooked	250	1400
Beef, uncooked	280	55
Corned beef	140	950
Haddock, uncooked	300	120
Haddock, smoked	190	790
Cabbage, uncooked	390	7
Cabbage, boiled	130	230
Horseradish, raw	564	8
Horseradish, prepared	290	96
Asparagus, raw	310	2
Asparagus, canned	250	200
Peas, fresh	380	1
Peas, frozen	135	115
Peas, canned	96	236
Peas, canned (served with ½ oz salted butter)	99	374

Adapted from the following: McCance and Widdowson's *The Composition of Foods*, 4th ed., A.A. Paul and D.A.T. Southgate (New York: Elsevier/North-Holland Biomedical, 1978); *Dietary Goals for the United States*, prepared by the staff of the Select Committee on Nutrition and Human Needs, United States Senate, February 1977 (Washington, D.C: U.S. Government Printing Office, *1977); Nutrition Almanac*, John D. Kirschmann (Minneapolis, Minnesota: Nutrition Search,1973).

See the problem? Even haddock, a salt-water fish, naturally contains nearly two-and-a-half times as much potassium as sodium. But when turned into a more easily-preserved and tastier treat, the ratio of the two minerals becomes almost four-to-one in the wrong direction. And your body is asked to deal with a food environment that is very different from the one for which it was designed. Almost all whole foods start with potassium outweighing sodium by a far larger ratio. But after the processors, packagers, and cooks have finished their work (not to mention what may be added at the table), this relationship has been drastically altered, and in many cases reversed.

The interaction of certain minerals is one of the major factors affecting whether or not your body will use, lose, store, or abhor a particular mineral. Interdependencies of nutritional significance (to researchers' knowledge at present) include:

> *sodium-potassium*
> calcium-magnesium
> manganese-iron
> iron-copper
> zinc-copper

These proportions become detrimental to your wellbeing when the first metal of each pair listed is available in too large an amount, while the other is at the lower limit of your dietary requirement.[6]

There are a tremendous number of ways in which today's modern food milieu subjects you to similar differences, forcing situations and substitutions completely foreign to your metabolism. Most of these transformations do not work in your favor. But this book focuses on one particular change — the amount of potassium in your food and its outcome on your sodium-potassium ratios. Understanding the far-reaching effects this has on human health — on *your* health — is a recent event. Suggestions for positive action to correct this problem are noted in these chapters, including simple *dietary changes* and/or safe *potassium supplementation.* (Given today's lifestyle, the latter may be the easiest recourse for many.)

WHY YOU SHOULD CARE

Should you care about your potassium and sodium levels? The most common answer to this question is, "Yes — because of high blood pressure." Sodium and high blood pressure, or *hypertension*, have been linked together for so long that nearly all educated laypeople are aware of the connection, at least in theory. You've heard it and read it again and yet again: "People with high blood pressure should cut down on salt."

You have also heard of some sort of controversy — that perhaps your body will *only* be unhappy with your salt consumption if you are among the 10 percent of people who are salt-sensitive. But the problem of sodium excess, which in turn affects potassium metabolism, is more complicated. *There are far-reaching health ramifications when sodium and potassium are not in balance, in addition to those related to hypertension.*[7]

Checking for the salt/blood pressure correlations during the day may not tell you the total story. Salt restriction tends to have more of an effect during resting and sleep pressures. During waking time, when compensatory mechanisms are involved, it may have a lesser effect. So the timing of varying research protocols may be responsible for the salt-hypertension controversy. Some researchers suggest that the culprit is the chloride in the salt.

American Journal of Public Health, 1991[8]
The Nutrition Report, 1991[9]

Potassium deficiency — or, more accurately, potassium deficiency in relation to sodium quantity — has been associated with many disorders, either as cause or effect. These include the following:

accelerated aging

acne

alcoholism

anorexia

antibiotics[10]

blurred vision

cancer

chronic fatigue syndrome

cognitive impairment[11]

cold sensations

constipation

depression

diarrhea

diabetes

EKG alterations[12]

edema

enlarged heart[13]

fatigue

gastric slow-down

glucose intolerance

growth impairment

headaches

heart arrhythmias[14]

hypertension

increased heart rate[15]

insomnia

low blood sugar[16]

intolerance to cardiac drugs[17]

kidney damage

muscle cramps

muscle tics

muscle weakness

nausea

nervousness

neurological disorders

osteoporosis

rapid pulse

respiratory problems

salt retention

sensation of cold

short stature

slow sperm motility

stroke[18]

suppressed immune system

surgery[19]

tear duct/gland dysfunction

tingling sensations

weakness and lethargy

You probably have some personal experience of at least a few of the problems cited — conditions you or those close to you may have known. This is not surprising if you eat a "normal" North American diet. It would be extraordinary if you *hadn't* ever suffered from one or more of these afflictions. That most of us manage as well as we do for as long as we do is testimony to the incredible adaptability of human physiology — a shift of function, resorting to the use of reserves, as explained in the Prologue, which takes place as your enzymes and neurons spread a plea for help. None of us, however, should be too smug about the apparent ease of this adjustment. Just as you can feel or be ill in the absence of disease, you can also have disease and not feel ill. Hypertension is an example of the latter. Most diseases, unfortunately, start on a cellular level, very quietly, and unannounced. By the time symptoms blow the whistle, the damage has often been done.

Two-thirds of Americans over 60 have high blood pressure. When hypertension-free individuals from low salt cultures adopt a higher salt diet, blood pressure begins to rise.

American Journal of Clinical Nutrition, 1988[20]

It is not unusual for symptoms of potassium excess to be similar to those of potassium deficiency. Too much or too little of the same nutrient often results in parallel ailments. In the case of potassium, either disorder may even be life-threatening.

I have a fantasy — initiated because I know we cannot "hear" the beginning stages of an illness. In my dream, every time we consume highly processed foods, our body cells would respond *instantly* — as though the non-nourishing foods were explosives! We'd surely have a world full of very noisy and different dining tables.

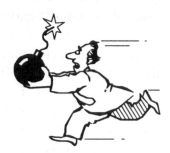

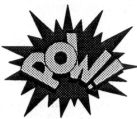

This would call attention to the earliest initial roots of the disease state, otherwise unnoticed. Unfortunately, whether we're talking about temporary indigestion or extreme allergic sensitivity, whether the food eaten causes a minor impairment or leads to serious conditions, these symptoms often remain dormant for a period of time before surfacing.

Disease occurs naturally; diagnoses are artifacts. Potassium deficiency may exist despite normal serum potassium levels.[21]

Age and Aging, 1984

WHAT IS POTASSIUM?

(A very small amount of required chemistry, necessary for understanding preventive medicine.)

Potassium is an element. That means it occurs as an atom, one of the basic chemical building blocks that make up a molecule. Hydrogen, oxygen, carbon, sodium, calcium, sulfur, iron, or aluminum are also elements, and also occur as atoms within molecules. In fact, there are about 109 elements, but only about 45 are known to have any significance in human nutrition. Of these 45, only about 30 are considered essential to human health — to the best of current knowledge.

Groups of atoms bonded together into molecules are described as "compounds". Sugars, starches, fats, proteins, vitamins, and plastics are different types of compounds. Molecules can be made up of just two or three atoms or can also be very big, and there are myriad numbers of such possible combinations of elements.

The 109 elements are numbered according to weight, starting with the lightest, which is hydrogen. Potassium is number 19, which means there are 18 elements that are lighter than potassium, and about 90 which are heavier. A very fundamental building block for many common substances, potassium as a fairly light element is quite simple compared with some other nutritionally-important constituents. Large molecules like fats, sugars and carbohydrates consist of many atoms linked together in an infinite variety of geometric variations. Proteins can be enormously complex. The information contained in a single DNA protein molecule, which is a miracle of organization in the way it dictates your genetic inheritance, challenges the limits of human comprehension. But potassium is simple: 19 protons, 20 neutrons, and 19 electrons.

What makes potassium interesting is its nineteenth place on the element chart. It seems that 18 is one of those "magic" numbers of chemistry because it is the number of electrons which forms a stable electron "cloud." Modern chemists prefer not to use the term "orbit," although this may have been the designation you were exposed to in school. Argon is the very stable element with 18 protons and 18 electrons. (Because nothing reacts with argon, it is called one of the *inert* elements.) But potassium has one more proton and one more electron. This last electron is out by itself in a new region of the electron cloud. It is very easily removed from association with the potassium atom, requiring relatively little energy for this to happen — making potassium an element which is quick to react, or bond, with another element.

Sodium has the same property. With 11 protons and 11 electrons, sodium's place on the element chart is one above another magic number: the number 10, also a stable configuration. (Neon is the inert element with 10 protons and 10 electrons.)

When potassium and sodium are dissolved in water, they are good at conducting electricity. Electrical current is simply the flow of electrons. *The solo "outer" electrons of sodium and potassium can move freely from atom to atom.* So it is that they share the property of being able to conduct electricity easily when dissolved. In fact, solutions into which these elements (or other charge-carrying particles) are dissolved are called *electrolytes* — liquids that conduct electricity. In human metabolism, electro- lytes figure heavily in the function of both potassium and sodium.

One more thing about potassium and sodium: because they are both so reactive, each with its one extra electron, they are usually combined with other elements when in solid form. Chlorine, for example, has only 17 electrons — one short of the magic number 18. There is a "space" in the electron cloud caused by a missing electron. So chlorine loves to accept an additional electron while potassium and sodium love to give one up. The resulting "charged" atoms or "ions" have a very strong attraction for each other, like north and south poles of magnets. The two atoms have a fondness for locking together, almost like the "hooks" and "fuzz" of velcro. Think of the extra electron from the sodium or potassium atom *filling the slot* for the "missing" electron around the chlorine atom when the atoms pair up, or "bond". Now both atoms "think" they have 18 electrons.

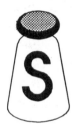

Sodium chloride, the molecule resulting from the attraction between sodium and chlorine is another name for table salt. Potassium combines with chlorine in the same way to form *potassium chloride*, another kind of salt.

Dry table salt will not easily allow electricity to pass through it (that is, conduct electricity). When table salt is dissolved in water, however, it dissociates (breaks down) into freely floating sodium and chlorine ions. The solution can now be called an "electrolyte".

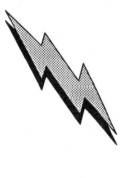

As for the chemistry, we'll try not to get any more technical than the presentation you have just read.

POTASSIUM, SODIUM, AND CELL MEMBRANES

(Now for a little biology, and a touch of electrical engineering.)

No matter if you don't fully understand the following few pages. Reading through the explanations and looking at the diagrams starting on page 37 should help you to grasp the *concepts*, if not the details.

Every living thing more complicated than a virus is composed of cells — the microscopic compartments of tissue in which most of the real work of biological processes takes place. The hurly-burly pace of New York City is sedate when compared with the activity within every one of these trillions of units. But not only is each cell a microcosm in itself, with a life of its own, each cell participates in dense interrelated communities whose maneuvers are ceaseless — even when you sleep.

Tiny and numerous as they are, cells communicate, accommodate, collaborate, negotiate, and replicate. Each consumes energy and manufactures proteins, enzymes, and hormones. Every cell generates waste products, regulates its own growth and reproduction, and has wonderfully intricate ways of blocking the entrance of harmful, unwanted foreigners — while absorbing what it *does* need and want.

Your genetic code is embedded in each cell in the form of a huge DNA molecule (huge, that is, compared with other molecules), which directs all the cell's activities, including metabolism and self-duplication. It is awesome to think of these complex events occurring in cells that are invisible to the naked eye.

Blood plasma or lymphatic fluid is outside the cell membrane and is the medium in which all cells are bathed. Cytoplasm is on the inside, the cell's internal fluid. One of the most intriguing parts of each of these already-Lilliputian cells is the diminutive thinness of its membrane — the boundary between the outside of the cell and the cell's interior, between the blood plasma and the cytoplasm.

The membrane is only two molecules thick, but performs an amazing number of control and guardian functions. These relate to the regulation of what goes in and what comes out of the cell, with the membrane acting as both ticket-taker and bouncer. Visualizing the size of a cell and its jam-packed activity is forbidding enough. Attempting to grasp the image of the mere wisp of its membrane wall, boasting all these distinguished achievements, is even more extraordinary. But as we zero in closer and closer, we actually get an expanded view of how we function!

So we see that membranes are *smart* and membranes *work hard,* size notwithstanding. They consume a good deal of energy in order to move substances in and out, often against the natural tendencies of these materials to proceed in the opposite direction. More than that, they transport atoms and molecules selectively in ways that support very complicated processes within the cell.

In fact, one of the primary functions of nearly all cell membranes is to keep sodium out and let potassium in. This function alone has been estimated to consume *one-third* of all the energy that comes from your food and is used by your body.[22] One-third! There must be something very important about keeping sodium out and holding potassium in. And in fact there is. The difference in sodium concentration between the outside and inside of your cells can be thought of as an engine which in turn drives a multitude of other membrane functions. This single energy-consuming process — facilitated by the proteins in the cell membrane — powers this engine. The process is often referred to as the *sodium-potassium pump.*

Here's how the sodium-potassium pump works: (See Figures 1 to 7) Whenever two potassium ions on the outside of the cell come in contact with a certain protein in the cell membrane at the same time that three sodium ions on the inside happen to come in contact with the same protein, chemical energy is consumed to push the three sodium ions out of the cell, allowing the two potassium ions to enter. Remember that all the atoms here have lost that extra electron when they dissolved, so we say they have a positive charge of +1, which means each is set up to attract a single electron to fill the gap. After the membrane protein completes its work, three atoms have gone out (sodium), and two have come in (potassium). Many repetitions later, there is significantly less positive charge inside the cell than outside because of the 3-to-2 exchange. (One positive charge is lost with each sodium-potassium exchange.) The difference in voltage between the inside and the outside of the cell can actually be measured using tiny electrodes.

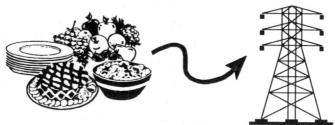

Look what you've done: You've converted chemical energy (initially supplied by your food) into electrical energy!

Now what happens? It turns out that most cell membranes are relatively permeable to potassium but will not let sodium through except as a result of special reactions — when the sodium-potassium pump is triggered, as described above. That is, potassium can move both in and out easily, a process that can be thought of as *dissolving* (actually, diffusing) through the membrane. But once sodium is pushed out, it stays out. Potassium ions, however, are attracted to the cell (opposite electrical charges attract; similar charges repel). Or, more accurately, the potassium ions are *repelled less* by the *inside* of the cell than by the *outside* of the cell. It's as if the cell interior is at the bottom of a hill, and movement away from the cell in any direction is like trudging uphill. Moving toward or into the cell is like sliding down hill — much easier. At least that's how it looks to a positively-charged potassium ion.

So the potassium "rolls down" to the inside of the cell through cell wall. But, for each new potassium ion that comes in, another positive charge is added to the interior of the cell. This tends to reduce the relatively negative charge of the interior.

Won't the cell eventually "fill up" with new positive charges, and stop when its charge equalizes with the charge on the exterior? Isn't it like water coming to the same level on two sides of a leaky dam? No, because the electrical attraction is only one of two forces involved. The other force is caused by something called the *concentration gradient,* which also affects the rate of diffusion in and out of the cell. If there were no electrical forces involved at all, potassium would diffuse in and out of the cell freely until its concentration inside and outside were the same. (A balloon with a leak will eventually reach the pressure of the outside air.) However, when the concentration of potassium inside the cell is high, and the concentration outside the cell is low, it's as if the interior of the cell were now the top of the hill. Potassium tends to roll "down" the concentration gradient, from high to low, moving to the outside of the cell once a certain concentration is reached inside.

The result is a balance between the force pulling the potassium in (electricity) and the force pushing it out (concentration). Eventually a balance is reached — an equilibrium between the *concentration gradient* and the *electrical potential* created by the sodium-potassium pump. Because of the balance, there's lots of potassium but very little sodium inside the cell. Outside the cell, however, there's a great deal of sodium and very little potassium. In fact, concentrations of potassium are normally 40 times greater inside the cell than outside.[23]

THE ROLE OF CALCIUM

A very important process which depends on the relationship of sodium and potassium is the regulation of calcium levels inside the cell. (See Figures 8 to 11) Calcium is a key factor in muscle function. In the muscles which comprise the walls of arteries, for example, the amount of calcium determines how much these muscles contract, and how much they relax. If there is too much calcium in the cell — *even by a small margin* — the muscle cell will not fully relax in response to the appropriate nerve or chemical signal. When there's a fairly high concentration of calcium outside the cell, and only a little bit in the interior, removing calcium from the cell requires moving it in the "uphill" direction. And this requires energy. In addition, a calcium ion has a charge of +2. That is, there are two electrons that leave the atom when it dissolves in solution. So the calcium ion is strongly attracted to the relatively negatively charged region of the cell's interior, and even more energy is needed to get the calcium out of the cell. This attraction has twice as much force as the attraction of a potassium ion, with its charge of only +1.[24] (As you have probably experienced, a magnet with twice the magnetic charge will stick twice as hard to the same refrigerator.)

What the cell membrane does is capture three sodium ions from outside the cell (with a combined charge of +3) and exchange them for one calcium ion). Letting these three sodium ions enter results in the release of electrical energy — more than the electrical energy required to push the calcium out, and with enough energy left over to overcome the concentration gradient as well. This is how the membrane can push the calcium "uphill" to where there is both a higher concentration of calcium and a strong electrical repulsion force. In this case the membrane doesn't have to do any work — the energy is taken from the electrical potential already built up by the sodium-potassium pump. But the membrane still has to be *smart* to do this at the right time!

You may already be recognizing some clue as to why potassium is so important. Without an ample supply of potassium in your plasma between your cells, cell membranes cannot generate the electrical difference across their cell boundaries, which in turn restricts the membrane's ability to remove sodium from the cell's interior. The sodium will back up in the cell like cars on a freeway on a rainy day. Remember, it takes potassium ions on the outside to remove sodium from the inside. If sodium can't be removed, the voltage difference across the cell membrane will drop. And if this voltage drops, processes such as the control of calcium levels can't run at full power. You then compromise the efficiency of fully one-third of the total body energy you consume. No wonder that people with low potassium levels are always so tired! And it should be no surprise that diet change or a supplement addition which increases potassium in safe amounts helps to reduce fatigue. Wouldn't you prefer to use your energy for more useful or more fun-filled endeavors than for inefficient cellular functions?

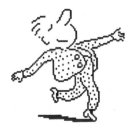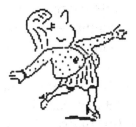

Efficient
potassium
metabolism

Inefficient
potassium
metabolism

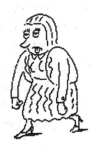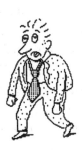

Too much sodium does the same thing as too little potassium. In the presence of excess sodium, it becomes more difficult for the membrane's sodium-potassium pump to find potassium because of all that sodium in the way. Too many empty shells and too few nuts! Consequently, the same result ensues, as above.

The processes involved — meant initially for your survival in a world that once upon a time offered high potassium and low sodium — are no longer always in your best health interest, given the eating patterns of contemporary society.

If you don't understand all the details, take heart. You can be an excellent driver without comprehending all the intricacies of the internal combustion engine. Again — it's the general *concept* that's important. A small moment of clarity is all that is necessary.

Regardless of what reason you had for picking up this book in the first place, there is probably some secondary condition that you'll find unexpectedly improved — just because you are beginning to pay attention to potassium and change your habits. Addressing this most fundamental of health concerns has myriad benefits.

> Any nutrient that stimulates normal biological activity, while interrupting abnormal chains of occurrences (without drug use), almost always has multiple gains.

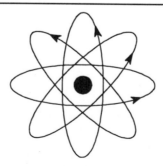

EXPLAINING THE SODIUM-POTASSIUM PUMP

This is where potassium plays its most important role — at the cell membrane. The sodium pump powers a wide variety of cell membrane processes and may consume as much as one-third of your total food-energy supply to do this.

The next 11 pages show how it works:

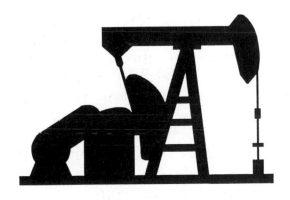

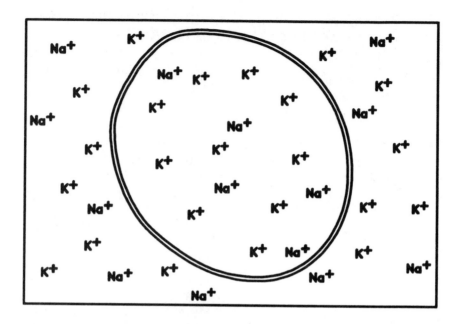

FIGURE 1

This is a typical cell, with the cell membrane forming the boundary between the inside and outside. For our purposes, we'll imagine an unrealistic
initial condition in which the sodium and potassium ions are distributed evenly inside and outside
the cell. Na+ is a positively-charged sodium ion,
and K+ is a positively-charged potassium ion.

This is a close-up of part of the cell membrane, showing the sodium-potassium pump protein. This large protein molecule attracts sodium on the inside of the cell membrane and potassium on the outside of the cell membrane.

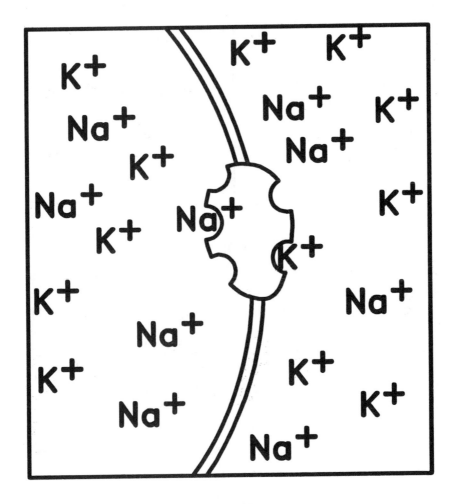

FIGURE 2

The protein has receptacles to accept three sodium ions and two potassium ions.

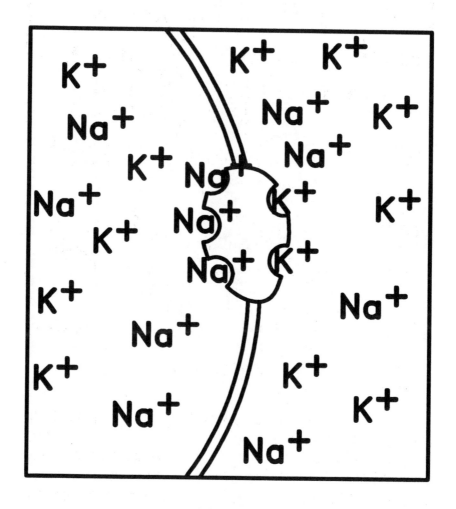

FIGURE 3

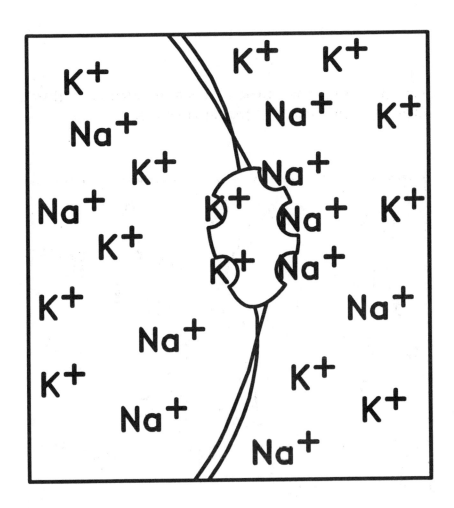

FIGURE 4

Then the protein inverts itself, pulling the sodium ions out and pushing the potassium ions in. After this process has gone on for a while, the protein will have to work against electrical potential because there will be less positive charge on the inside and more on the outside. Chemical energy is used by the protein to move the ions through the membrane against this force.

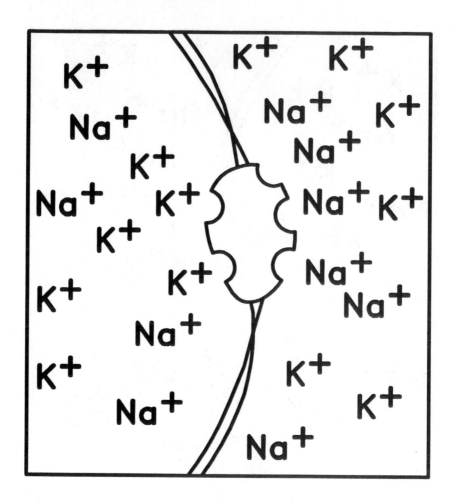

FIGURE 5

The protein releases the sodium outside the cell, and the potassium inside the cell.

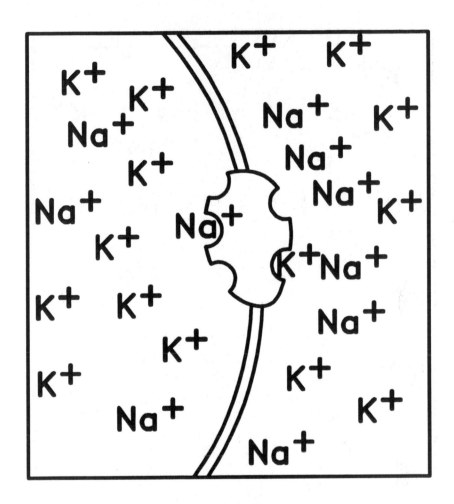

FIGURE 6

Now the protein flips back, and is ready to repeat the sodium-potassium pumping process. But because there is less potassium outside, and less sodium inside, it takes longer for the protein to pick up the ions for pumping.

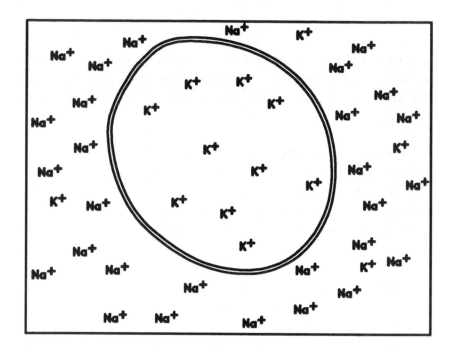

FIGURE 7

This is what the cell looks like after the sodium-potassium pump has done its work. Sodium, outside, and potassium, inside. But because the exchange is two-for-three, there is a net reduction in positive charge inside the cell.

Similar electrical charges, like similar poles of magnets, tend to repel each other. Every positively-charged ion is repelled by every other positively-charged ion, so they are pushed to where the concentration of positive charges is the least. The result is that all positively-charged ions are now strongly attracted to the interior of the cell.

Calcium-flow in and out of muscle cells is one example of a membrane process that is powered by the energy stored by the sodium-potassium pump.

Calcium ions (depicted here as Ca++ because they have an electrical charge of +2) enter the cell when the muscle contracts. They are strongly attracted to the inside of the cell, so no energy is required to let the calcium ions in.

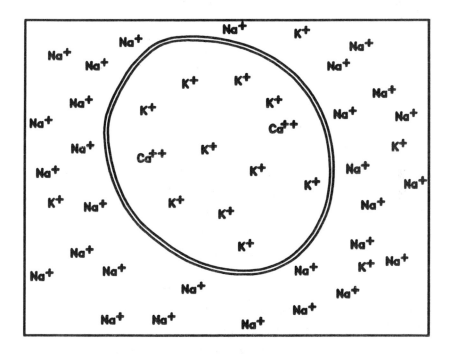

FIGURE 8

For the muscle to relax, the calcium must be removed. This is accomplished by other proteins in the cell membrane, which let three sodium ions in for every calcium ion that they push out.

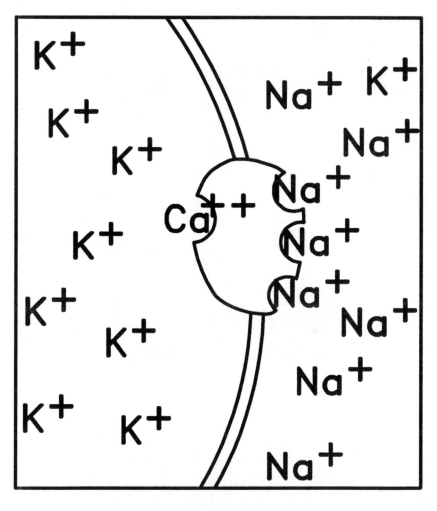

FIGURE 9

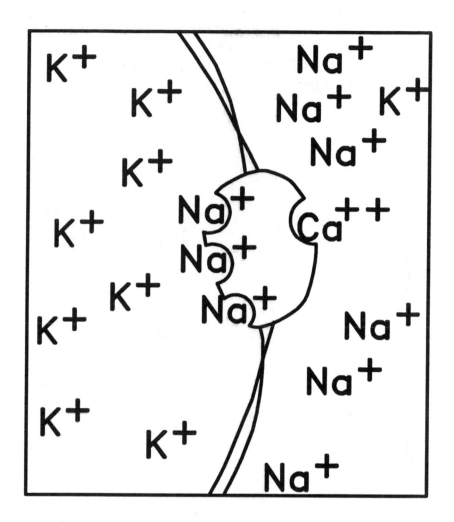

FIGURE 10

Because three sodium ions with a total charge of +3 are attracted to the inside of the cell even more than is one calcium ion with only a charge of +2, no additional energy is required for this exchange to take place, and the calcium can be quickly removed.

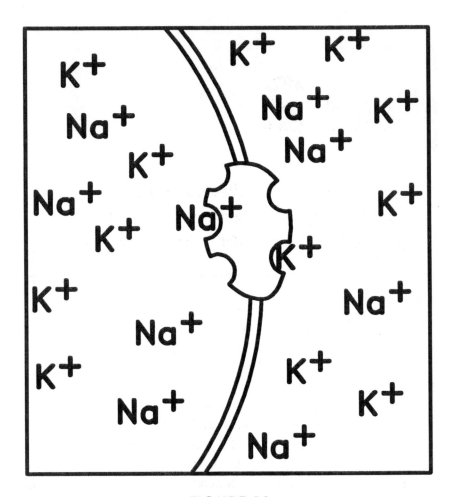

FIGURE 11

However, this process has depleted some of the energy stored by the sodium-potassium pump when the sodium was allowed back into the cell.

More potassium must be available for the pump to remove the sodium and restore the cell's supply of electrical and chemical energy.

PART 2

*in which we discuss why it is
that not getting enough potassium
affects your health and life quality.*

POTASSIUM DEFICIENCY

Neither our wonderful physicians nor medical science can be very much credited for wiping out the dreaded infectious diseases that plagued us into the early years of this century. The real heroes are those who made it possible to prevent these diseases: engineers who improved water conduits; economists who improved living conditions; agriculturists who improved food availability; inventors who ingeniously created diagnostic and surgical tools. But we have traded infectious disease (with a few very serious exceptions) for degenerative disease. Who will be our next heroes?

Joseph Califano, Jr., past Secretary of Health, Education, and Welfare, points to America at the dawn of the first four-generation society in the history of the world. "That dawn," says Califano, "can be the start of a brilliant era in which great-grandfathers pass on a rich, living inheritance of love and wisdom to their great-grandchildren." Then he adds: *"Or it can be the beginning of a frightening era of death-control."*

One panel of experts estimated that 90 percent of America's health status is determined by factors over which doctors have little or no control. The Commission on Critical Choices for Americans concluded that we are "doing better and feeling worse."

I can only point out: there has never been a time when more people were aware that they can be responsible for their own health. Our new benefactors guiding us toward the best ways in which to do such preventive self-care may be the science researchers and/or the nutrition educator, acting as intermediaries—teaching every-one—including the doctors—how to make our own bodies the real heroes!

Even when medical researchers are "onto" something in today's high-tech, high-media world, it can still take almost a lifetime for the information cited in the journals to filter through to the average practitioner — given the double-blind studies and the large number of participants necessary for official acceptance of new discoveries (to say nothing of the money and politics involved). The most important and up-to-date research information as to how best to preserve and improve your health is very often not widely available; the information which most doctors and patients have access to is all too often out of date and may even be inaccurate.

Sodium-potassium metabolism is a disturbing case-in-point. The medical literature is actually chock-full of associations between the faulty functioning of these two minerals and human disorders. But awareness of these correlations on the part of practicing physicians or the food industry are not common. Research also is clear concerning the value of potassium supplementation, a prescription often not recommended for the right reasons, if at all, and certainly not frequently enough. This section explores potas-sium deficiency and its impact on health. Once again, recall that no discussion about potassium deficiency is complete without including sodium excess.

POTASSIUM, SODIUM, AND BLOOD PRESSURE

If, at around age 40, you meet with three of your friends for a school reunion, chances are that only one of you will have "normal" blood pressure.

Three in four at age forty fail the
"Perfect Blood Pressure" test.

For the other three with higher levels, risks of seriously impaired well-being and reduced life quality are markedly increased. The strong links between high blood pressure and health hazards trigger secondary events that continue to have deleterious consequences in more ways than are commonly assumed.[1] The reason: hypertension is not a disease, but an indicator, a risk factor. Cardiovascular risk, for example, is directly proportional to the level of your blood pressure.[2]

Even more alarming is the fact that the danger involved is sizable not only for persons testing high by the usual criteria, but also for those with "high-normal" blood pressure levels.[3]

You have high blood pressure if:
 • your systolic pressure is greater than
      or equal to 140
 • your diastolic pressure is greater than
      or equal to 90
You have high-normal blood pressure if:
 • your systolic pressure is 130-139
 • your diastolic pressure is 80-89

memo:

"Because we have deserted our ancient cuisine (high potassium and low sodium), we have helped to produce diseases of civilization, including hypertension. Studies indicate that a 'normal' potassium diet can prevent many arterial and renal lesions, even though blood pressure remains hypertensive. The use of a high potassium diet is a prime example of protecting arteries in a hypertensive setting. This is a new dimension in hypertension therapy — protecting the arteries."

Clinical and Experimental Hypertension, Theory and Practice, 1992[4]

THE ROLE OF CALCIUM IN HIGH BLOOD PRESSURE

The control of calcium as outlined in Part I is just a single example of how a vital cell process is powered by the sodium-potassium pump. Many other illustrations of the critical importance of its role exist, and they probably relate to more health conditions than we know about. But the calcium connection is particularly significant because of its effect on your circulatory system — the system that circulates blood and lymph throughout your body.

Arteries, the blood vessels that carry blood to all of your body tissues, are more than just passive runs of piping. Arteries have muscles in their walls for controlling diameter and elasticity. They do this by means of varying the tension in the artery wall (hence the term *hypertension* for high blood pressure). This muscle control can be likened to a garden hose. Control the pressure at the end of the hose by manipulating the opening of the nozzle. The stream of water can be forceful, or diffused and "soft."

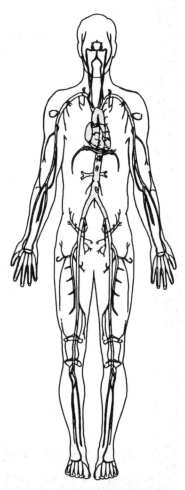

ARTERIAL SYSTEM

Why should it be necessary to vary the diameters of these passageways? Isn't there a powerful pump forcing blood through all the tributaries which loop through your body? Yes, but the problem is that there are many thousands of routes for blood to take after it leaves your heart. Let's assume that all tissues require an equal flow of blood. No biological system could possibly be so perfectly symmetrical as to allow the blood to flow equally through all the branches in your body without some active control.

The process is not unlike pouring gravy on a plate piled high with mashed potatoes. No matter how carefully you pour the gravy on top of the potatoes, the gravy will not run down evenly on all sides — even if the pile of mashed potatoes is perfectly round. Some of the potato will be covered with gravy, some will be dry. No matter that it's all downhill from the source at the top to every point on the surface of the potatoes. There are so many ways for the gravy to flow down and nothing to direct the flow evenly.

Blood flow is similar to the gravy pouring over the mashed potatoes. What we want would be the equivalent of a thin film of gravy spread evenly all over the mound of potatoes — equal flow through all the branches of your circulatory system. The muscles in your artery walls contract and relax with each heartbeat and also in response to the more slowly-varying changes in demand. This is what insures sufficient blood flow to all parts of your body and to all tissues. So your arteries are not just pipes — they need to be *smart* and work *smart*.

HEART VALVES

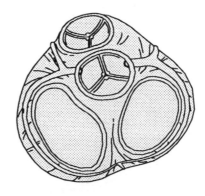

The sodium-potassium pump also facilitates the movement of calcium in and out of muscle cells, as explained in Part I. To summarize: not enough potassium, or too much sodium, and cell membranes find it more difficult to remove calcium quickly. Calcium removal — in fact, extremely rapid calcium removal from the muscle cells — is part of the process that induces these cells to relax. If there is too much cellular calcium:

- arterial muscles cannot fully relax
- the average artery size diminishes
- your heart has to work harder to move the same amount of blood
- your arteries become less elastic, which causes turbulence in the blood flow and results in damage to the cells lining the inner walls of your arteries

Now you know the basic relationship between low potassium and high blood pressure — not enough potassium, or too much sodium, and the calcium levels in the muscle cells of your arteries are likely to be too high. Consequently, arteries don't work the way they should, and your blood pressure goes up.[5]

Surprisingly, a low amount of calcium in your blood does not have the effect of reducing the problem of high calcium. It seems that if calcium levels outside the cells are very low, the cells conserve calcium instead of pumping it out. It's somewhat analogous to behavior during a gasoline shortage. When gas is hard to get, you tend to get your car tank filled whenever you can and you keep it filled. Chances are you'll "top" the tank every time you pass a gas station.

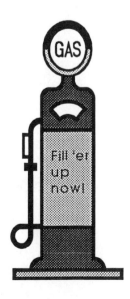

So even though calcium appears to be one of the culprits in hypertension, it's only an intermediary. True, you do need a generous supply of calcium. But getting enough calcium can be deceptive. The amount of calcium consumed is frequently different from the amount of calcium absorbed. Then, too, calcium supplementation itself can be tricky business. There is a tremendous amount of misinformation passing for common wisdom. For example, did you know that milk is not conducive to good calcium absorption (especially *low-fat* milk)? Avoiding sunshine totally can interfere with calcium metabolism? Too much exercise depletes calcium reserves? Eating meat reduces calcium absorption? (To learn more about factors that help or hinder calcium absorption, you may want to check out my inexpensive booklet, *Startling New Facts About Osteoporosis.*)

The absorption of dietary calcium requires the presence of fat.[6] Among the factors 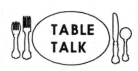 influencing proper calcium absorption are foods ingested in the same meal. Foods that enhance the absorption of calcium are fatty fish (like salmon), eggs, butter, and liver. Foods that diminish the absorption of calcium are sodas, unleavened bread, and milk.[7] (Yes, and milk! Trust me!)

Of interest to women approaching menopause: Total body potassium is significantly related to total body calcium and the bone density of your spine and radium.

American Journal of Clinical Nutrition, 1991[8]

(See the list of high-potassium foods on page 116, and/or consider a safe potassium supplement, as outlined in Part III.)

SODIUM AND HIGH BLOOD PRESSURE

Yet another mechanism contributes to high blood pressure. Your kidneys remove excess sodium, but, as cited in Part I, kidneys are not very efficient at accomplishing this job. Your body is much better at removing potassium (which, as stated, is far more abundant in a natural diet). Sodium must diffuse out of your blood as it passes through your kidneys. This diffusion is driven at least in part by blood pressure, so if your blood pressure increases, more sodium can be removed.

In other words, high blood pressure is, at least temporarily, a proper and desirable response to excess sodium, caused by constriction of the peripheral vascular system (the smaller and more numerous blood vessels). It's as if more pressure, very simply, is forcing more sodium out of your blood.

> Potassium citrate provides excellent therapy for those who are excreting too much calcium because this form of potassium reduces abnormal calcium excretion.
>
> *Journal of Urology, 1989*[9]

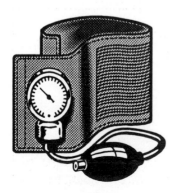

As stated so eloquently by Dr. James Scala, "Elevation of blood pressure to eliminate more sodium shouldn't surprise anyone with engineering knowledge."[10]

Explanations presented here should offer a better understanding of why risk factors include high salt intake and a high dietary sodium-potassium ratio — that is, a diet comprised of more sodium than potassium.[11] The natural safety measure of your body to reduce sodium by increasing pressure works to your health advantage — as long as it doesn't get out of hand.

Leg symptoms can be a condition especially related to hypertension.

Western Journal of Medicine, 1991[12]

WHY *EVERYONE* SHOULD RESTRICT SODIUM

Again — controversy abounds as to whether or not salt restriction should be recommended to everyone. A few studies show that only 10 percent of the population may be dangerously sodium-sensitive. But note these points:

(1) Biological measurements are never black or white. You may be at least somewhat, if not fully, sensitive to salt. There is little likelihood that all those "at risk" will be identified.

(2) Sodium deficiency is no threat because more than enough is present in natural foods, and far too much pervades processed foods.[13] There is no known hazard to sodium restriction. But such restriction will benefit the salt-sensitive subset. If we include people who are partially sensitive, the total adds up to a significant majority — certainly far more than 10 percent.

(3) The effect of salt intake on your sodium-potassium ratio is highly significant in other disease states — even if it doesn't affect your blood pressure.

(4) A study reported in *Hypertension* in 1991 shows that a dietary deficiency of potassium amplifies the effect of a high salt intake on your blood pressure.[14]

(5) If you are potassium-deficient and do not restrict your sodium intake, and then you take a potassium supplement, the additional potassium has only a moderately hypotensive effect.[15] (However, any positive consequences, even in modest amounts, should be gratefully acknowledged.)

(6) An extraordinary review called, "High Blood Pressure: Hunting the Genes," emphasizes the fact that, although we do not yet know which genes are involved in high blood pressure, environmental factors such as salt intake could influence the rate or timing of the expression of the genes which lead to this disorder. Such genes have been located in test animals.[16] *The influence of the environment on gene function is more and more apparent.*

When population studies are made within a homogeneous country like the United States, they show a major connection between increasing dietary salt intake and higher blood pressure.

No negative consequences of reducing salt intake have been observed, and in some cases improvement in the dietary intake of *other* nutrients occurs when salt is reduced.

British Medical Journal, 1991[17]
Hypertension, 1991[18]

VALIDATING THE SODIUM-POTASSIUM/ HIGH BLOOD PRESSURE CONNECTION

Here are some studies which validate the sodium-potassium/high blood pressure concepts outlined in this section:

➤*Clinical Science*, 1992: A low level of the sodium-potassium pump activity is associated with high blood pressure.[19]

➤*Circulation*, 1992: Variations in potassium levels may contribute to sudden cardiac death in those with hypertension.[20]

➤*Journal of the American College of Cardiology*, 1991: Even modest potassium depletion within what has been considered a "low-normal" range can impair the contractile and relaxation responses of certain heart functions.[21]

➤ *Journal of Microscopy*, 1991: An imbalance of potassium in cardiac muscle causes an alteration of heart function.[22]

➤*American Journal of Medicine*, 1991: Blood pressure decreases with a decline in sodium intake, which, of course, alters the sodium-potassium ratio.[23]

The continuous wear and tear of muscle pumping and a marginal nutrient supply can gradually weaken your heart's pumping ability.

My doctor told me to jog for my health. When I told him I already do, he said, "In that case, you'd better give it up!"

➤*Journal of Cardiovascular Pharmacology*, 1990: The World Health Organization Cardiovascular Diseases and Alimentary Comparison Study demonstrates that decreased salt and increased potassium consumption are effective measures for blood pressure reduction even in those over 65.[24]

➤*American Journal of Hypertension*, 1990: The sodium-potassium ratio in your cells tends to be higher if you have hypertension.[25]

➤*Journal of Human Hypertension*, 1990: A high sodium-potassium ratio is positively correlated with high blood pressure, but potassium appears to be the more important component of this ratio.[26]

➤*New England Journal of Medicine*, 1989: Potassium depletion in normal individuals causes sodium retention and increased blood pressure.[27]

➤*American Journal of Clinical Nutrition*, 1981: Every population that adds little or no salt to its food ends up with little or no rise in blood pressure, while every population that adds a half teaspoon or more of salt daily sees blood pressure escalate as people grow older.[28]

➤*Reference to Clinical Nutrition: A Guide for Physicians*, 1979: Excess intake of sodium, which may result from the ingestion of some commercial baby foods, may predispose infants to hypertension in later life.[29]

Given the odds, salt reduction makes sense!

Your body adapts well and likes a low salt, high-activity lifestyle. It's your biological heritage.

HYPERTENSION AROUND THE WORLD

Comparing populations within a community and between communities presents an opportunity to use the entire world as a laboratory. Note these observations:

➤*Cardiovascular Pharmacology*, 1990: Hypertension is a bigger problem in the capital city of Tanzania where the rate of obesity and salt intake are higher than in other parts of East Africa.[30]

➤*Journal of Cardiovascular Pharmacology*, 1990: In two Ecuadorian populations mortality from stroke is positively related to salt consumption.[31]

> It has been shown that conventional techniques such as diet history and interview studies in conjunction with standard food tables do not provide the true intake levels of trace elements from prepared meals.
>
> *Biological Trace Element Research*, 1989[32]

➤*Annali di Igiene*, 1989: A study was carried out in the Italian Marches Region in which food habits were examined and analyzed. The food was sampled ready for consumption so that it had already undergone various preparation and cooking procedures. The researchers wanted their results to include the changes in mineral content which occur during these processes. Among the conclusions: the presence of a high sodium intake, and thus a high sodium-potassium ratio, has been associated with hypertension risk.[33]

➤*Journal of Hypertension*, 1987: The variation of sodium excretion within-person and between-person is smaller among Chinese men than among American men, showing that the range of sodium intake by Americans is very much broader.[34]

memo:

A report related to heart disease in general (not just hypertension specifically), and issued about thirty years ago by the L. Peter Cogan Foundation of New York, showed that national heart disease rates are inversely tied to potassium in a nation's traditional foods. Where potassium-rich foods are frequently consumed (Japan, Scandinavia, Italy, France, Germany, Netherlands and Switzerland) the heart disease rates are low, compared with countries whose diets are not rich in potassium (United States, Australia, Canada, New Zealand, United Kingdom).

The Japanese eat plenty of potassium in seafood and seaweed (kelp), and in mushrooms used frequently in their national dishes. Italians are also fond of seafood. Olive oil, grape wine (both good potassium sources), and vegetables are part of every meal.

HYPERTENSION AND INDIVIDUAL DIFFERENCES

The same guidelines cannot be used for all people when determining blood-pressure risk. Matching for race, sex, stage of menstrual cycle (in women), family history of hypertension, and the amount of sodium in your diet must all be considered.[35]

Note these ethnic and sex variations:

• Hypertension is more common and more severe in African Americans than in the white population of the United States.[36] Compared with whites, many normotensive healthy blacks (those whose blood pressure is neither too high nor too low) have more sodium in their cells due to an inherited depressed activity of the sodium-potassium pump.[37] Symptoms at the same blood-pressure level are also more severe in blacks.[38] Evidence points to one biologically relevant explanation: an inherited tendency to accumulate heavy metals (environmental toxins, like lead and cadmium) in the cells.[39] To confuse the issue, blacks are *less* likely than whites to get osteoporosis — but there is a potassium-metabolism tie-in with this disease.

• In healthy women, the sodium concentration in certain cells is lower during particular phases of the menstrual cycle. This adaptation helps to explain deviations between men and women.

• Women have been generally excluded in widespread testing demonstrating the adverse effects of antihypertensive agents.[40]

Researchers suggest that "the ultimate goal of further knowledge in the area of heart health should be to understand the fundamental abnormalities responsible for hypertension. Such insight would permit more effective treatment and, perhaps, primary prevention of the ubiquitous and multifaceted disorder."[41] And that's one of the objectives of this book!

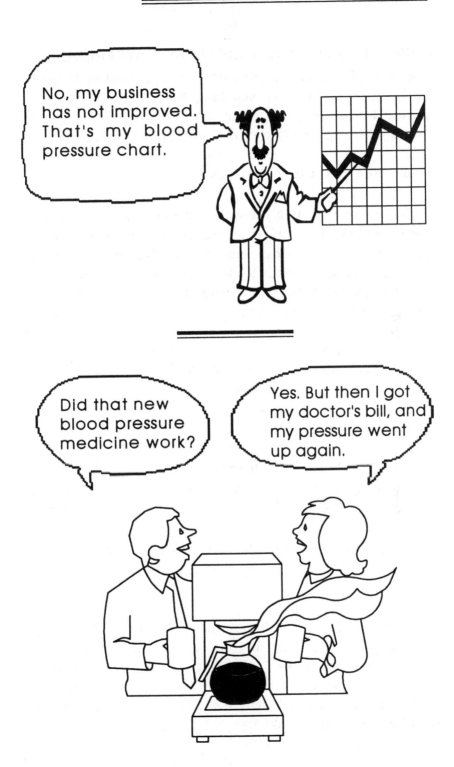

HYPERTENSION DRUGS AND SIDE EFFECTS

Because hypertension may be a "silent" disease, getting patient compliance with therapy is often a problem.[42] Isn't it true that those in pain are more inclined to take their medicine? But, actually, serious concerns regarding blood pressure medications do center around their side effects.

As many as 10-to-15 percent of patients (that we know about) withdraw from high-blood-pressure therapy because of undesirable side effects.[43] Combine this with the increasing appreciation that the majority of those with mild blood pressure elevations have not derived cardiac benefits from drug therapy![44] Drugs that lower blood pressure often leave the real problem unresolved. One group of drugs — angiotensin-converting enzyme (ACE) inhibitors — is now known to have been prescribed in doses that were inappropriately high. Dose-related adverse effects were observed frequently.[45] What side effects will surface after the new drugs have been in use a few years?

The fact remains that high blood pressure is population-wide, and there is no consensus among the experts concerning the best treatment program. Nor is there agreement for the treatment of mild hypertension: Should lifestyle changes alone be used, or should this treatment include a pharmacologic component?

The difficulty is accentuated by the availability of a plethora of blood-pressure-lowering drugs. Five classes of agents, including angiotensin-converting enzyme inhibitors, beta-blockers, calcium-entry blockers, peripheral alpha-1-adrenergic receptor blockers, and thiazide diuretic agents, are all on hand now. The doctor must be astute enough to make the right choice for each patient — no easy task.[46] Once you start hypertension therapy, you must be monitored by your physician on a regular basis. It is also difficult to separate disease effects in hypertension from true drug effects.[47]

Many physicians believe that the health risks of some drugs used to treat mild hypertension outweigh the marginal benefit that patients in this group (who may not even have hypertension) would obtain.[48] Even diuretics have been criticized recently because of a substantial number of significant side effects.[49]

> The Oslo Study shows that hypertensive men on medication do not live as long as those not taking medication.
>
> *Nutrition Research Reviews*, 1990[50]

During the last five years, community-based studies from Dalby, Gothenburg, and Glasgow have reported a high risk of cardiovascular (especially cardiac) disease, even though these hypertensive patients have been well-cared for and their blood pressure controlled. Long-standing hypertension may cause irreversible cardiovascular change and atherosclerosis — which contribute to increased risk even when elevated arterial blood pressure has been reduced to normal levels. According to these researchers, another possible explanation is that the antihypertensive drugs themselves, while they have a blood pressure-lowering effect, have adverse effects. By elevating serum lipoproteins or by *lowering serum potassium*, some drugs could increase the risk of cardiovascular complications and, to a certain extent, offset the advantages of lowering blood pressure.[51]

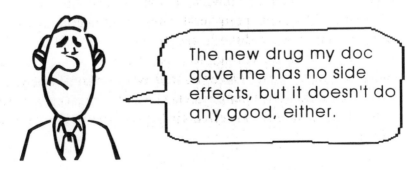

The new drug my doc gave me has no side effects, but it doesn't do any good, either.

Commonly used hypertensive drugs can cause:

• impaired exercise performance (propanolol, beta-blockers)[52,53]
• increased sexual problems in men, affecting life quality[54]
• fatigue, by compromising sodium-potassium pump activity, resulting in inhibition of ion movement between muscle and plasma (beta-blockers)[55]
• dry mouth (transdermal clonidine)[56]
• skin reactions (transdermal clonidine)[57]
• dry cough[58]
• deterioration in glucose control, not only in the general population but especially in those with impaired glucose tolerance (thiazide diuretics)[59]
• disturbed sodium metabolism (thiazide diuretics)[60]
• depression[61]
• gastrointestinal symptoms such as nausea and disturbed intestinal motility[62]

More than 16,000 people were studied in an effort to determine the effects of non-drug intervention on blood pressure. The results were reported in the *Journal of the American Medical Association,* March, 1992. Neither stress management or the use of ordinary multi-type supplements reduced high blood pressure in those with high normal levels.[63] Unique supplements (those with high bioavailability), coupled with dietary changes? That's another story.

Another more recent controlled trial, reported in the *Journal of Human Hypertension* in June of 1991, confirmed that drug treatment has side effects, and may be associated with increased cardiovascular risk not found with dietary alternatives.[64]

Those interested in this concept may find remarkable non-drug therapeutic results for hypertension by following suggestions outlined in Part III. Discuss these with your physician.

memo:

This commentary on diet and blood pressure appeared in *Hypertension:*

"Use of dietary measures as sole therapy for hypertension has generated enthusiasm and is supported by data. Dietary measures should be effective in preventing the rise in blood pressure with age. Weight loss and sodium restriction may be of benefit to the drug-treated patient.

"There are strong reasons to consider the use of nonpharmacological measures for the treatment of mild hypertension, which is ubiquitous. A high proportion of the population is in need of drug therapy. If a change in lifestyle could reduce this need by a respectable percentage, then an enormous number of individuals could be spared the necessity of taking antihypertensive medication."[64]

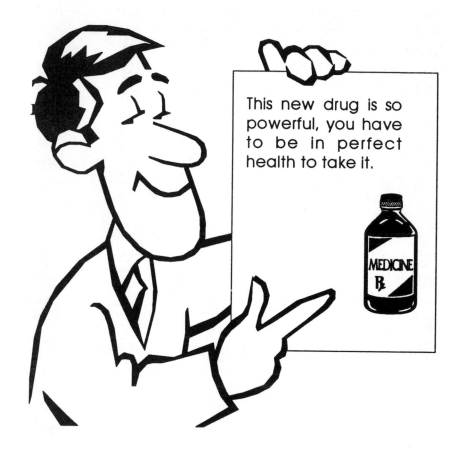

POTASSIUM AND FATIGUE

OVERVIEW

Are there times in your life when you feel left out of the world? Perhaps you go through the day's paces wishing you had more energy? Surely these are feelings we have all experienced. Judging from interviews with physicians, plus articles and books in the popular press, fatigue appears to be increasing in prevalence and duration. Two physicians give interesting accounts of patient experiences:

➤ Dr. Robert Cathcart of San Mateo, California, describes some of his chronic fatigue patients as being so tired that they must rest on the floor en route from bed to bathroom. This may appear extreme, but most physicians who treat patients with chronic fatigue syndrome relate similar stories.

➤ Dr. Michael Rosenbaum of Corte Madera, California, describes a patient whose serum potassium level was 3.1. Since 3.0 suggests a medical crisis (normal levels are between 3.5 and 4.5), it was no surprise to Dr. Rosenbaum that this patient was suffering from chronic fatigue. What is surprising, however, is the oversight of standard physicians regarding potassium metabolism. This particular patient had seen two other physicians, neither of whom raised an eyebrow when checking her potassium chemistry. According to Rosenbaum, potassium levels are 50 percent reduced before they are even seen in a blood test. (It took less than a month to get the patient's levels back to normal, and for her fatigue to vanish.)[66]

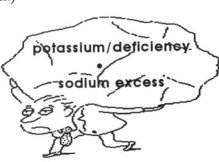

THE ATHLETE, FATIGUE AND POTASSIUM

Athletes have been among the first to recognize potassium as a critical nutrient in fatigue prevention. By studying athlete/fatigue responses, we learn a little more about potassium and the general population.

When muscle tissue is tired, the concentration of potassium in the extracellular fluid around muscle cells goes up, not down. So an accumulation of potassium ions in the extracellular space is associated with fatigue — a good signalling mechanism, according to several researchers.[67,68,69] Why, then, would an athlete want more potassium? What's going on?

The increase in potassium around muscle cells is a direct result of potassium diffusing out of these cells as the electromotive force across the cell membrane decreases. Remember that this voltage difference across the cells drives multiple reactions — among them the transport of calcium in and out of muscle cells to control the contraction and relaxation of muscles. When the cell is working hard, the sodium-potassium pump can't keep up.

Calcium enters cells easily because the +2 charge of the calcium ion pushes it towards the relatively negatively-charged cell interior. But when the calcium needs to be removed for muscle contractions or relaxation, remember that three sodium ions with a total charge of +3 have to be let in for each calcium ion that is pushed out. This transaction reduces the difference in the electric potential between the inside and outside of the cell, which in turn reduces the cell's next response to the positively-charged calcium. This loss of response in turn means that the sodium-potassium pump can't keep up with other reactions as well that draw on this stored energy. The muscle cell "gets tired." Some experimenters have demonstrated a voltage drop of as much as 50-percent across cell membranes in fatigued muscle tissue.

When muscle activity stops, the cell recharges. Potassium slowly returns to the cell interior, and the sodium-potassium pump eventually removes most of the sodium that had to be let in so that the calcium could get out.[70,71]

Other factors such as lactic acid and carbon dioxide also play a major role in muscle fatigue.

The high extracellular potassium level may also be part of a signalling mechanism, telling the appropriate nerves that the cell is tired.

In order to keep muscle cells fully "charged up" before activity, the sodium-potassium pump has to have access to an ample concentration of potassium before the exertion begins. And after exertion, an "electrolytic replacement" drink may be useful to restore potassium lost through perspiration. Because of prolonged losses of potassium from the skin through sweat, athletes are likely to have higher potassium requirements than sedentary people. But an on-the-spot potassium dose won't instantly extend the fatigue limit. It might, however, improve recovery time before the *next* exertion — more so if heavy perspiration is involved. Studies of the effects of fluid intake during an ultramarathon running race show that they do not change serum sodium or potassium.[72]

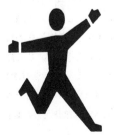 An important point for the athlete: a potassium dose has an effect on *future* exertions.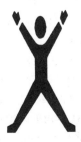

Additional facts:

➤Muscle tissue is the main reservoir of potassium.[73]

➤The site of exercise-induced muscle fatigue appears to be the muscle-cell membrane.[74]

➤Intense muscle contractions result in large changes in the concentrations of electrolytes, including potassium.[75,76]

➤The contraction-induced potassium loss may play a major role in muscle performance since it may impair mechanical force production, and it is hypothesized that this may be the origin of low-frequency fatigue. There is still a significant potassium deficit seen after one hour of recovery following voluntary contractions. Researchers conclude that potassium recovery is a slow process after prolonged low intensity contractions — due to inefficient sodium-potassium pump activation.[77]

➤The marked increase in blood levels of potassium during maximal exercise coincides with leg-muscle fatigue.[78]

Muscle potassium loss has been cited as a major factor associated with or contributing to muscle fatigue.[79]

American Journal of Physiology, 1992

People used to work out; now we work in, so we have to work out.

But — given the facts above, is exercise a good idea? Yes, as the next section explains.

HOW EXERCISE REDUCES FATIGUE

The loss of potassium decreases with continued exercise and training. This may be one reason why we feel better when we exercise regularly.

That's good news for the exerciser and, perhaps, an incentive for the non-mover to get going.

Here are some interesting excerpts from a study reported in the *European Journal of Clinical Investigation*, 1990:

➤Loss of potassium from the skeletal muscle pool during exercise is reduced after training.

➤Your heart during exercise may be exposed to a smaller rise in plasma potassium concentration after training than before.

➤Moderate improvement of your capacity to clear extracellular potassium during exercise results in processes that reduce muscle fatigue and also increase physical performance.[80]

Other studies confirm that strenuous short-term exercise has a beneficial antihypertensive effect and has a favorable outcome on plasma potassium homeostasis.[81]

And yet another interesting report resulting from experiments with test animals shows that potassium supplementation reduces heat-distressed consequences.[82]

These studies emphasize the reasons why daily exercise is so important. *Seniors*, take note: The percent of improvement with exercise is similar in all age groups! *Everyone*, take note: Daily moderate exercise partially postpones the ravages of aging!

We appear to come back to square one, no matter what the research or the subject: *Watch your diet, take your supplements, and exercise.* Easier said than done — the reason for Part III!

FLUID INTAKE DURING EXERCISE?

The optimum fluid for rehydration during exercise depends on many factors, particularly the intensity and duration of the exercise, environmental conditions, and individual physiology of the athlete. Note that:

- there is no advantage to fluid intake during exercise of less than 30 minutes duration
- the addition of potassium is important for rehydration after more lengthy exercise[83]

What about sodium for the exerciser? An hour of vigorous exercise in hot, humid weather could result in a sodium loss of 2,000 milligrams. For typical American eaters, 3,000 to 6,000 milligrams of sodium daily is not unusual. You only require a minimum of 115 milligrams of sodium a day, and athletes can probably get by on less than 500 milligrams daily. So the chances of ending up with a sodium deficit, even after two hours of profuse sweating, are next to none.

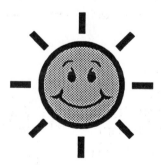

It is believed that athletes following low salt diets produce more salt-retaining hormones, and do not suffer salt depletion. But potassium is a *must* when exercising in warm weather.

CHRONIC FATIGUE

There are many suspected reasons for chronic fatigue, and it is not known what fraction of these might be caused by potassium deficiency. It is known, however, that deficiency of dietary potassium does cause chronic fatigue. As indicated, chronic (but not acute) changes in potassium concentration are significantly correlated with changes in your energy expenditure.[84]

As early as 1962, clinical researchers were reporting success with potassium in the treatment of chronic fatigue. And now there is intriguing new evidence that potassium supplementation is very effective in alleviating this condition for a greater percentage of people than previously believed. A few relationships follow.

Fatigue and Epstein-Barr
(also known as recurrent mononucleosis)
Between 35 and 80 percent of students entering college will test positive for Epstein-Barr antibodies. Another 10 to 15 percent will become infected during their first year, an equal percentage during their second year, and so on. At age thirty, 97 percent test positive! *The one symptom that shows up in 100 percent of Epstein-Barr cases is fatigue.*

People who react to daily activities as though they were difficult chores, and plough through or postpone activities they enjoy, often test positive for active Epstein-Barr virus.

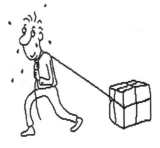

A recent article in *Biochemical Pharmacology*, 1992, describes the metabolism in certain cells which have been transformed by the Epstein-Barr virus. This includes a reduction in the extracellular concentration of potassium, causing changes in the number and activity of sodium-potassium pumps in the cell membrane.[85]

Fatigue and your adrenal glands
Potassium helps your adrenal glands. Here's how:

➤There are immunologically active substances found in the adrenals and controlled by the sodium-potassium pump.[86]

➤Potassium intake has been shown to direct the manufacture of certain adrenal enzymes.[87]

➤The adrenals manufacture renin, a substance important in calcium metabolism. Renin secretion is regulated and stimulated by potassium.[88]

➤Adrenal regulation is helped by dietary sodium depletion or potassium intake.[89]

What does this have to do with fatigue? Chronic stress can deplete your adrenal glands to the point of exhaustion. In his book, *Solving the Puzzle of Chronic Fatigue* , Dr. Michael Rosenbaum says:

> Chronic fatigue syndrome puts relentless strain on the adrenal glands. Theoretically, chronic stress can deplete the adrenal glands to the point of "adrenal exhaustion." The nutritional management of this adrenal exhaustion can make a huge difference in how a chronic fatigue syndrome patient ultimately responds.[90]

How your adrenals respond to certain secretions remains unclear, but we do know that potassium is a major factor in regulation, and that its control is of considerable importance.[91]

Annual Review of Physiology, 1988

Fatigue and environmental pollution

Sometimes the loss of electrolytes is the first warning signal of metal toxicity. Heavy metals like cadmium, mercury and methyl-mercury inhibit sodium-potassium activity.[92] Other contaminants cause different dramatic changes and may increase their transport in a nonfunctional manner.[93] Nickel and lead cause more pronounced losses of potassium than sodium, a balance bound to be off-ratio already![94]

The impact of low-level lead exposure on the human central nervous system function has become a major public health concern. The average blood level of lead in the United States is high enough to impair important human brain function. Studies show that the sodium-potassium pump is affected by lead.[95]

(See page 85 for Dr. Hans Nieper's theory on catalytic converters in automobiles and chronic fatigue syndrome.)

Fatigue and hidden malnutrition

Dr. Jesse Stoff, in *Chronic Fatigue Syndrome: The Hidden Epidemic*, states:

> To strengthen the vital systems of the body (the liver
> and associated immune defenses), we must use simi-
> larly vital therapies.

"Vital" therapy translates to foods and/or supplements that are nutrient-dense.

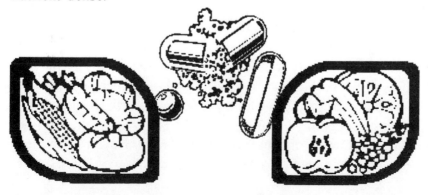

POTASSIUM AND AGING

Did you think you would ever be old or tired when you were a teenager? And isn't it equally as difficult to think of yourself as middle-aged when you are only forty? As cited in the Prologue, many silent aging changes occur on your way to becoming "senior." Some of these, like skeletal bone loss, are initiated very early. As for the adaptation of your kidneys to sodium, *the descent begins in your thirties.*[96]

There is an age-related decline in sodium-potassium-enzyme activity. The older you are, the less efficient the activity.

Mechanisms of Aging and Development, 1991[97]

AGING AND GROWTH HORMONE

Remember the story of *The Princess and the Pea*? The princess was accustomed to luxury. Her true identity was revealed only when she complained about her mattress resting on a pea. Now a particular secretion of a pea-sized gland has people agog at the prospect of maintaining a more youthful image. The pituitary, located on the underside of your brain at the level of your eyes, is considered a master gland because it controls many other glands. But the pituitary itself is powered by your hypothalamus. And among its goodies is a fountain-of-youth elixir, *growth hormone.*

According to a study done at the Medical College of Wisconsin in Milwaukee, the reduced availability of *growth hormone* is a major contributor to making you look and feel old, but the decline of this hormone starts in your thirties.[98] You can imagine the flurry of excitement with this breakthrough news! Haven't we been searching for a magic youth potion for all of recorded history?

Because synthetic growth hormone had already been in place for medical applications (mostly administered to undersized children), attempts to use it as an anti-aging potion spread like wildfire. But the results have not been very promising. Among the side effects of synthetic growth hormone:

- adverse carbohydrate metabolism (producing too much insulin, glucose intolerance, and diabetes)
- unfriendly musculoskeletal metabolism (initiating arthritis and arthralgia)
- cardiovascular performance problems (leading to hypertension, edema, and congestive heart failure)[99]
- depleted bank balances (produced by the high cost of growth hormone)

Nutrition plays a major role in the production of growth hormone. I conducted an extensive world-wide database search to obtain information on what foods to eat and what not to eat — an effort to find determinants for the natural assembly of our own growth hormone. My endeavors produced only a handful of very general reports. Among the information that surfaced was this gem:

There is a correlation between the reduction in growth hormone and the reduction of dietary potassium.[100]

So potassium just might help to stave off accelerated aging! (What else is new!)

Aging and potassium balance

How do we age? We can count endless ways, but let's describe one: In the event of too much or too little potassium, a single cell becomes nonfunctional, and you are one cell older. No matter, you have trillions of other cells — your body will hardly know the difference. But another cell is compromised, and you are two cells older. Then three! Four! And more! Eventually, tissue is affected. Finally, an organ. Now it matters. Now your body notices. *As you lose cellular efficiency, so you age.*

Here are the results of studies demonstrating the relationship between decreasing potassium (or increasing sodium) and aging:

➤*Journal of Membrane Biology,* 1991; *Fiziologicheskii Zhurnal,* 1990: The permeability of cells to potassium declines with age.[101,102]

➤*Clinica Chimica Acta,* 1991: Differences between young and old in the sodium-potassium pump rate is even more marked in those who are frail.[103] (Older people are more likely to be frail.)

➤*Life Sciences,* 1991: Because the reserve capacity of the sodium pump drops with age, there is a diminished margin of safety against digitalis toxicity.[104]

➤*American Review of Respiratory Disease,* 1991: Dietary potassium has an influence on airway responsiveness in middle-aged and older men. This is an important consideration since respiratory problems increase with aging.[105]

➤Both sodium and potassium activities have the same characteristics in certain cell membranes throughout the life span of the animal, but they decrease quantitatively with aging.[106]

➤*Clinical and Experimental Hypertension,* 1990: The sodium content of diets is found to increase with advancing age.[107]

➤*Clinical Chemistry,* 1987: Research underlines the large prevalence of magnesium and potassium deficiencies in the elderly, an observation that could not be attributed to pathology or treatment.[108]

➤*American Medical Association,* 1969: A study at the University of Glasgow determined that a decrease in muscular strength, usually accepted as a symptom of "old age," may have been simply a lack of potassium in the diet.[109]

> Old age is the most unexpected of all the things that happen to a [person].
>
> Leon Trotsky, *Diary in Exile*, 1935

The dreaded malady of aging, Alzheimer's disease, is *systemic* — it is not restricted to the central nervous system alone. The nature of Alzheimer-related changes in cells confirms and emphasizes the involvement of cellular membranes in this disease. Analysis of membrane changes in the cells of Alzheimer patients suggests that the normal aging process of these cells is disturbed.[110] Inadequate function of the sodium-potassium pump could be a major factor.

Another very common condition associated with aging is *xerostomia*, or dry mouth. At least one in five older adults suffers from this uncomfortable dilemma. Problems of lubricating, masticating, tolerating, tasting, and swallowing food contribute notably to the complex physiological and psychological manifestations of aging. Xerostomia is, therefore, a major contribution to the high prevalence of geriatric malnutrition in the United States. *More than 75 percent of seniors suffering from xerostomia were shown to have significant deficiencies of potassium, among other nutrients.*[111]

High blood pressure, fatigue, and aging are generally considered as separate entities. They are, however, very much related — as are the disorders described below. In other words, hypertension can impact on fatigue, aging influences high blood pressure, neurological problems may be tied to aging, and so on. The big lesson we've learned in recent years implicates an interaction of *all* parts and functions — connections we are only just beginning to understand. The head bone *is* connected to the neck bone.

POTASSIUM AND OTHER CONDITIONS

NEUROLOGICAL DISORDERS

Nerve cells send signals throughout your body by transmitting electrical impulses. But it's not a purely electrical process — there are links in the chain where electrical signals are converted to chemical signals, and then back again. Rather than contracting and relaxing, like a muscle cell, a nerve cell works to convert these various signals and pass them along. The electromotive force behind these signals comes from the sodium-potassium pump on the nerve-cell membrane. It's perfectly reasonable that potassium deficiency can have a devastating effect on your nervous system.[112]

Potassium deficiency is frequently associated with a restless and/or tearful mood — a general feeling of malaise. Decreased intracellular potassium has been noted in depressed patients. Those who have committed suicide have been found to have decreased cerebral potassium.[113]

These studies demonstrate how the sodium-potassium ratios affect various nerve responses:

➤*Developmental Brain Research*, 1991: Maintaining specific potassium concentrations in brain extracellular fluids is critical to proper neuronal function. Active potassium transport by certain cells in your brain plays an integral role in cerebrospinal fluid.[114]

➤*Journal of Hypertension*, 1991: Increased sympathetic nervous system activity is a well established feature of arterial hypertension. The researchers stress that attention to diet is mandatory, and include advice to augment potassium intake.[115]

➤*Brain Research*, 1991: When your sodium-potassium pump is not behaving properly, central nervous system neuropathology could be one of the serious consequences.[116]

➤*FASEB Journal*, 1990: The clinical signs of neuropathy in zinc deficiency are associated with decreased sodium-potassium activity of nerves.[117]

➤*Neuropsychobiology*, 1989: Values for sodium-pump activity are significantly lower in certain manic-depressive groups than in controls, and higher than normal in others.[118]

Sailors have related tales of insanity from drinking sea water in desperation when fresh water supplies were depleted. This represents an extreme example of changing electrolyte concentrations in your body and brain. The high salt content of sea water has a dehydrating effect.

STRESS

Dr. Hans Selye is associated with clarifications pertaining to stress. Among his numerous studies, he subjected test animals to severe stress, damaging heart muscles. This caused the animals to die prematurely. A control group which was given magnesium and *potassium* lived in spite of the stress.

Several biochemical changes, including sodium-potassium pump alterations, precede the appearance of stress ulcer.[119] It is also known that adrenal regulation is helped by dietary sodium depletion or potassium intake.[120] (See segment on "Fatigue and Adrenals," earlier in this chapter.)

As Horace said 2,000 years ago, "*Chase nature out, and she will return with a pitchfork.*"

BRONCHITIS

This is an oldie (but not so golden). Although chronic bronchitis was first named and described in 1808, the disease has been known since earliest time, and is *still* annoyingly prevalent. In Greek medicine, bronchitis was appreciated as one of "excess phlegm." Early remedies included garlic, pepper, cinnamon, and turpentine, whereas later therapies of choice emphasized coffee, ipecac, and potassium nitrate.[121] Why a potassium supplement? Bronchitis has been associated with the sodium-potassium ratio, demonstrating that the balance between these two minerals may influence the occurrence of respiratory symptoms — independent of cigarette smoking.[122] (We now know there are better supplemental forms of potassium than the nitrate variety.)

Test animals infected with bronchitis have significant changes in their electrolyte composition, including decreased transport of sodium into cells across membranes, and decreased potassium.[123]

TOXICITY AND IMMUNE FUNCTION

Part of immunity at the cellular level involves keeping dangerous substances out of the cell (toxins) while allowing the entry of required substances (nutrients). Because the sodium-potassium pump indirectly powers many membrane reactions, there is an important link between potassium and immunity. A cell that has frail membranes due to insufficient electrical potential is a weak and vulnerable cell, and will have a hard time keeping toxic substances and dangerous viruses out.

The impact of low-level lead exposure on the human central nervous system has become a major public health concern. The average blood level of lead in the United States is high enough to impair important human brain function. *Studies show that the sodium-potassium pump is affected by lead.*[124] Surely this is just one example of a toxin affecting the sodium-potassium pump.

Hans Nieper, an internist who manages a very successful clinic in Hannover, Germany, contends that the catalytic converters on cars are responsible for much of our degenerative disease. These pollution devices are made of platinum, which produces three deadly gasses. Dr. Nieper cites statistics indicating that regions of the world where these devices are in use correlate with extensive disease. He indicates, for example, that chronic fatigue syndrome is nonexistent where there are no catalytic converters. The toxins released from the converters, Nieper confirms, break down *cell membranes*.

Dr. Nieper carries his theory one step further. He believes that even those who carry the HIV virus will not come to harm if their cells are sufficiently electrically charged.[125] While I'm not ready to endorse either of the above theories, I think they're interesting enough to pass along.

DIABETES

Potassium is closely related to diabetes disorders. Potassium:

- is intimately connected with the metabolism of sucrose by cell membranes
- is associated with the production of insulin by the pancreas
- has been shown to lower the blood sugar of diabetic patients

The last effect may be why some ingredients in fruit juice and broth help to revive people from diabetic comas. Dietary potassium-loading induces important modifications in glucose transfer.[126]

Cells of diabetic subjects (non-insulin-dependent) were found to have 15 to 20 percent reductions in sodium-potassium pump activity.[127]

WEIGHT

As the numbers on the scale rises, the sodium content of certain cells also increases.[128] Overweight people often don't consume foods conducive to good sodium-potassium ratios. It is highly probable, however, that a healthful diet which encourages weight loss alters that ratio for the better — thereby producing many health benefits.[129,130] Good sodium-potassium ratios offer more energy. If you burn more energy, chances are you'll lose more weight. So it's an amplified response, a positive feedback loop.

There is one caveat, however: Caloric deprivation decreases potassium levels and thereby, glucose and insulin efficiency. When potassium supplementation accompanies a diet, better insulin and glucose utilization are a bonus benefit.[131]

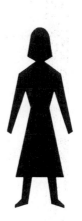

Adults on quick weight-loss diets show a 20 percent reduction of the enzyme activity controlling potassium and sodium metabolism in their red blood cells. And, as you now know, this depresses sodium-pump activity.[132]

Although weight loss is an important objective, how it is achieved is a critical factor.

memo:

Most people who are over-weight often experience *fluid-overload*. It's interesting to note that obesity is accompanied by an increase in the extracellular-to-intracellular fluid ratio — above that observed in nonobese people. Proper functioning of the sodium-potassium pump is important for weight maintenance because of its role in this ratio.[133] In both adolescents and adults, correlations between blood pressure and weight have been shown to be highly significant.[134]

So here's another incentive to cut back on salty snacks and increase potassium. There's more than just calories involved here.

ALCOHOLISM

If you've ever been to the emergency room of a hospital, you may have noticed that most of the people waiting for attention don't look healthy. Of course they don't — after all, they've just gone to the hospital. But you know what I mean: Do you think they looked healthy the day before or the month before? A significant percentage of emergency room patients are diagnosed as having alcohol or drug intoxication. What does this have to do with potassium? *Low levels of potassium have been associated with alcoholism, and even with intensity of symptoms.*

Potassium excretion will increase after alcohol ingestion. Alcoholics frequently exhibit potassium deficiency.

Many of the almost 300,000 sudden deaths that occur annually in the United States are related to alcoholism. Although the cause of sudden death in alcoholism is no doubt multifactorial, arrhythmias and stenosis have been implicated.[135] (Stenosis is the narrowing or contraction of the body passageways or vessels.) More than 150 years ago, Thomas Hodgkin wrote: "The heart and blood vessels do not escape the injurious effects of ardent spirits." Hodgkin's particular theories were confirmed in 1978 when a group of researchers described the "holiday heart syndrome." Patients in the study experienced a variety of symptomatic arrhythmias after drinking episodes.[136]

It is well known that potassium deficiency contributes significantly to arrhythmias associated with alcoholism.[137]

The sensitive potassium channels play a role in determining coronary responses.[138] One study demonstrates that arrhythmia susceptibility is reduced and onset delayed by raising the potassium concentration delivered to a certain coronary area.[139] Most arrhythmias result from malfunction of sodium channels.[140]

Potassium-sparing drugs have successfully reduced arrhythmias.[141] Agents that modulate cardiac and smooth muscle potassium channels have stimulated considerable interest in recent years because of their therapeutic potential in a number of cardiovascular diseases. But many of these agents suffer from a side-effect that is directly linked to their specific mechanism of action.[142]

The puzzle pieces are beginning to come together. Note the conclusions of the following studies:

➤*Veterinary and Human Toxicology*, 1991: Chronic alcoholics have lower serum potassium than non-alcoholics.[143]

➤*Journal of Neurology*, 1990: After correcting for potassium deficiency, alcoholic patients who have stopped drinking show complete recovery of neurological and neuropsychological function.[144]

➤*Emergency Medicine Clinics of North America*, 1990: There is no question about the presence of electrolyte abnormalities in the alcoholic patient.[145]

➤*Drug and Alcohol Dependence*, 1990: A close negative correlation between the intensity of alcohol withdrawal and serum potassium has been observed. Patients with delirium show lower levels of potassium at admission than patients without delirium.[146]

➤*Journal de Pharmacie de Belgique*, 1989: Variable daily doses (maximum 300 milligrams) of potassium administration result in a harmless and rather comfortable detoxification.[147]

➤*Circulation*, 1985: A low level of potassium is a predictor of arrhythmia.[148]

HEARING

High technology scanning devices have been instrumental in helping researchers discover more about the complexities of our hearing mechanisms. This equipment reveals that the activities of the sodium-potassium pump decrease significantly in the presence of intense noise exposure, and that this slack may contribute to a remarkable hearing shift (in addition to mechanical destruction by noise). *Metabolic disturbance may aggravate inner ear hair cell damage, leading to hearing loss.*[149]

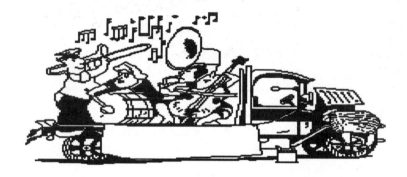

Other studies have also indicated an upheaval of sodium balance related to inner ear disorders.[150] Electrolyte imbalances may affect the inner ear, since *endolymph* (the fluid within the membranous labyrinth of the ear) is higher in potassium and *perilymph* (the fluid *between* the bony and membranous labyrinth of the ear) is higher in sodium.[151]

In Menière's disease, the increase of extracellular potassium concentration in the perilymph is thought to play a key role in the progressive loss of hair cells in the ear cavity. Cytotoxic activity affects the hair cells and auditory neurons as a result of this excess potassium *outside* the cells.[152] You may know Menière's as the disorder that causes progressive deafness, ringing in the ears (tinnitus), dizziness (vertigo), heightened sensitivity to loud sounds, headache, and/or nausea.

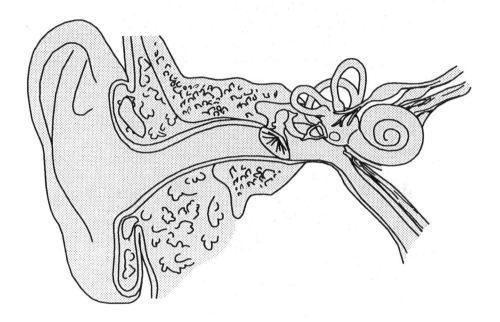

The hair cells of the inner ear work as electroreceptors, the outer hair cells as electrocytes. A layer of *potassium* ions on the lower surface of the membrane causes the excitation of the inner hair cells as soon as a certain contact occurs.[153] Again, when this metabolism is out of sorts, hearing troubles commence.

CANCER

The point being driven home here is that one of the greatest changes in the human diet has been the increase of the dietary sodium-potassium ratio — reported as being changed by a factor of about twenty. When I interviewed Dr. William Oliver, who studied the healthy Yanomama Indians in Brazil, he suggested that this factor may even be on the order of *100 to 200*. The primitive Yanomama do not eat salt but do grow and eat potassium-rich cooking bananas.[154]

Recall that humans initially had to adapt to retain sodium from a sodium-poor diet and to excrete potassium from a potassium-rich diet. We obviously have not yet reconciled (biologically) to today's high-sodium, low-potassium foods. As described in *Cancer Detection and Prevention*, and as you already know, this failure has caused increased rates of several diseases, *including cancer*. The influence of the sodium-potassium ratio on cancer development — first discovered by epidemiologic research — has been confirmed by various means, including:

- dietary studies
- gerontological studies
- studies of relationships between hyper- and hypokalemic diseases and cancer (that is, too much and too little potassium)
- review of cellular changes of this ratio induced by carcinogenic agents
- review of cellular changes of this ratio induced by anticarcinogenic agents
- animal experiments[155]

Research shows that the sodium-potassium ratio increases in test animals with tumors.[156,157] Other studies demonstrate that voltage-dependent channels may have an integral role in several small-cell carcinoma phenomena.[158]

Low consumption of salad vegetables and fruit (foods containing potassium) and the high intake of salt were clearly associated with stomach cancer development, as indicated in the *Journal of the National Cancer Institute*, 1989.[159]

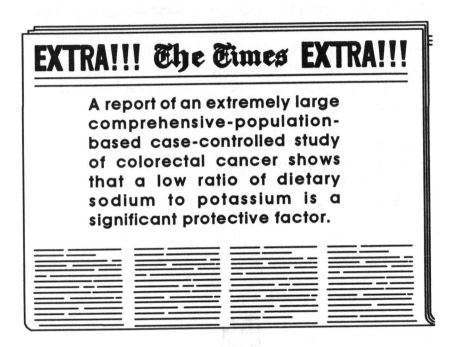

EXTRA!!! The Times EXTRA!!!

A report of an extremely large comprehensive-population-based case-controlled study of colorectal cancer shows that a low ratio of dietary sodium to potassium is a significant protective factor.

Since colorectal cancer is already epidemic in the United States, I think the results of this study (The Melbourne Colorectal Cancer Study[160]) should be front-page news. Shouldn't every physician be instructing patients at risk about how and what to eat to maintain a healthful sodium-potassium ratio? Or, for those who find lifestyle changes difficult, shouldn't they be told about safe supplements available which may help to achieve this goal?

Unfortunately, electrolyte disturbances cannot always be accurately predicted with our current testing equipment, even in high-risk patients.[161]

DIARRHEA

Potassium plays a fundamental role in the disturbance of electrolyte balance in the presence of diarrhea.[162] That's why Dr. Fima Lifshitz, Professor at Cornell University Medical College, states that traditional measures for checking diarrhea — such as fasting, and gradual resumption of diet with fluids and soft, bland foods — are not valid. Dr. Lifshitz says, *"The maintenance of electrolyte balance is vital."*[163]

ELEVATED CHOLESTEROL

Yes, even cholesterol enters the sodium-potassium picture:

➤*Experimental Physiology*, 1991: This study supports the hypothesis that there may be an optimum membrane cholesterol content for sodium pump function.[164]

➤*American Journal of Hypertension*, 1990: High potassium diets prevent hypertensive endothelial injury. By protecting endothelial cells, cholesterol-ester deposition can be decreased. This effect could possibly be useful for preventing atherosclerotic complications such as heart attacks in hypertension.[165]

➤*Journal of Hypertension*, 1989: Atherosclerotic cholesterol-ester deposition is markedly reduced with a high-potassium diet.[166]

Endless studies demonstrate that eating intact food containing cholesterol does not contribute to raised levels of cholesterol — and that includes eggs! If you are an egg-eater, try seasoning with a drop of tobasco sauce, which contains only 2.5 milligrams of salt, rather than salt itself.

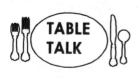
TABLE TALK

HEADACHE, ACNE AND OTHER MISCELLANEOUS PROBLEMS

No attempt will be made to explain the mechanism by which potassium deficiency may contribute to the conditions described in this section. They're not very well understood, anyway. But note the following:

Headaches

Headaches caused by certain allergies have been shown to respond well to potassium treatment. The associations of migraine headaches and potassium imbalances, among other mechanisms involved, were alluded to in one experimental study.[167] Substances which tend to lower hypertension are helpful for migraine. They work by possibly enhancing potassium-channel activations.[168] Headaches associated with Menière's, as cited in the section on hearing, are also relieved with improved sodium-potassium metabolism.

Acne

Both acne in adolescents and dry skin in adults are considered by some to be "a clarion call for more potassium."

Stroke

The risk of stroke decrease as the level of potassium increases, a process unrelated to blood pressure.[169]

Osteoporosis

Decrease in ability to retain electrolyte balance affects bone metabolism.[170] Low potassium intake increases urinary excretion of calcium and phosphorous.[171] Although association doesn't necessarily signify causation, it is more than coincidence that the rise in osteoporosis and other bone disorders have increased as potassium intake has decreased.

Colorectal polyps

A case-control study done in France shows that patients with colorectal polyps have a lower consumption of several important nutrients, including *potassium*.[172]

Tear function

A review of the ocular literature suggests that sufficient potassium, along with other nutrients (specifically, protein, vitamins A, B6, and C; and zinc) may be necessary for normal tear function.[173] The lacrimal gland is concerned with the production and drainage of tears — a protective device that helps keep your eye moist and free of dust and other irritating particles. Potassium is included in the nutrients which control the lacrimal gland output.[174]

Cataracts

Cataracts were induced in test animals, and observed prior to the onset of cataract formation. Among the results: the ratio of sodium to potassium increased.[175]

AIDS

Malnutrition in patients with AIDS is common and multifactorial.[176] Electrolyte disorders have been reported frequently in these patients. So has adrenal insufficiency. Diminished adrenal reserve and diarrhea both contribute to diminished potassium, hence electrolyte malfunction. We all know about the complexity of AIDS. Could the AIDS patient be helped with the addition of potassium? There are physicians who have had some positive results using special nutrient supplements, including potassium.[177] (We referred to Hans Neiper's theories on page 85.)

Check back to Part I, page 22, and look again at the disease states associated with potassium deficiency. After reviewing the studies in Part II, isn't it easier to understand why that list is so long?

POTASSIUM AND YOUR ACID-BASE BALANCE

Acidity or alkalinity is commonly expressed in "pH" units on a scale from 0.00 to 14.00. Anything above 7.0 is alkaline, and anything below 7.0 is labeled as acid. Acid/alkaline, or pH, are terms which refer to a condition created mostly by the food you eat. (Inherited tendencies and even mental attitudes also play a role.) Refined simple carbohydrates are generally more acid; complex carbohydrates may be more alkaline. Potassium is among the main alkalinizing minerals. (Calcium, magnesium, sodium, and iron are the others.)

A grade-school science teacher once taught a bit of mnemonics to help us remember the importance of the acid-base balance. He said: *A, B, C: acid-base-critical.* I never forgot that the ability of the body to maintain the blood pH within a very narrow range of about 7.4 was critical — necessary for life itself. *Potassium is crucial for this ongoing, vitally important process.* This is how it works: When your extracellular pH *decreases*, potassium exits from cells to bring your plasma level back up to normal. The reverse is true when extracellular pH increases. So the proper level is always secured! Well, almost always. In the presence of potassium deficiency and/or sodium excess there is a limit to how much defense takes place. The consequences frequently are suboptimal function and suboptimal health.

Some researchers believe that certain forms of cancer are accelerated by an acid condition of body fluids because cancer cells are able to live better than normal cells in an acid environment.[178] Even your nervous system and brain enter a slow-down mode when your blood leans to the acidic. Other forms of cancer have been demonstrated to relate to higher pH values.[179] Any value that deviates from the norm is not in your best health interest.

Serious acid-base disturbances are common in adults with alcohol intoxication.[180] The more we learn, the more the puzzle pieces fit: Chronic alcoholics have lower potassium than non-alcoholics, as explained earlier in this chapter.

POTASSIUM AND THE NEXT GENERATION

Let's start at the very beginning — with an overview of potassium and the life cycle.

INFERTILITY

Why are couples going off to Rumania and other foreign countries to find children for adoption? Part of the reason is that *the number of infertile women more than doubled between 1970 and 1985.* According to the National Center for Health Statistics, the increase continues to accelerate. Twenty-five percent of women in their thirties are infertile. That's one in four in this category, now a popular age for conception. More than nine million individuals are affected.

Note the following:

➤*Molecular Reproduction and Development,* 1991: Both the conservation and the regeneration of the sperm's capacity to move is dependent on potassium in test animals.[181]

➤*Presse Medicale,* 1990; *Journal of Obstetrics and Gynecology,* 1990: Imbalanced diets affect female fertility.[182,183]

➤*Journal of Dairy Science,* 1989: A borderline intake of several minerals may be detrimental to fertility.[184]

➤*Journal of Dairy Science,* 1989: *Potassium-deficient test animals show significantly reduced sperm motility.*[185]

➤*International Journal of Andrology,* 1989: An altered electrolyte milieu may be responsible for infertility.[186]

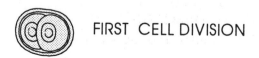 FIRST CELL DIVISION

PREGNANCY AND LACTATION

Totally overlooked in dietary advice to pregnant women is the fact that sodium deficits in the blood can also be caused by potassium deficiencies. You now know that when there is not enough potassium in the cell, the sodium in your blood may actually replace the potassium inside the cell. The low blood levels of sodium often observed in pregnant women do not necessarily mean a lack of dietary sodium, but could be indicative of a lack of dietary potassium. In studies that examine the effect of potassium deficiency on developing human embryonic kidneys, the results show abnormalities in the kidneys.

We have swung back to natural deliveries and natural feedings. Why not return to our natural sodium-potassium metabolism to insure the best possible health status for the next generation? I take strong exception to the "ob/gyn" physician who recommends increased salt for pregnant women. (If your doctor does make this suggestion, refer him/her to this book for a lesson in sodium-potassium nutrition.)

The more potassium-deficient the mother is during pregnancy, the greater the blood pressure of the child at age six months and twelve months.[187] As for the mother herself, the sodium-potassium ratio is positively associated with blood pressure during lactation and weaning.[188] The effect of potassium deficiency has been evaluated on growth and shown to have a negative correlation. The good news is that administration of potassium in infancy appears to reverse the effect of depletion.[189] Potassium supplementation for infants must be undertaken with extreme caution, however, and only under the direct supervision of a pediatrician. Indiscriminate use of potassium supplements is known to cause infant deaths.

WARNING: POTASSIUM SUPPLEMENTATION SHOULD NOT BE ADMINISTERED TO AN INFANT WITHOUT A PHYSICIAN'S PRESCRIPTION.

CHILDREN

Do we inherit genes or do we inherit diets? Usually both! An increase in sodium concentration and a decrease in sodium-potassium activity has been observed in the cells of offspring of hypertensive parents. Although there is a strong genetic influence contributing to these alterations, the influence of environmental factors should also be considered.[190]

The Food and Drug Administration's four-year *Total Diet Study* shows that sodium levels (which do not include salt added at the table) are significantly elevated for *two-year-old children* and teenage boys.

Journal of the American Dietetic Association, 1989[191]

The diets of younger children (but not older children), are related to their parents' diets — which, obviously, are more highly correlated with that of the parent in charge of meals.[192]

Australian six-year-olds in an urban area (not unlike so many neighborhoods in the United States) were checked for nutrient intake. Although their levels of potassium were adequate, those of sodium were high in relation to the recommended sodium-potassium ratio. A quick look at the salt content of junk snack foods can be very revealing.

A healthful dietary start is one of the best lifetime gifts you can give to your child. If you have young children, take advantage of your captive audience.

Children usually love corn on the cob. Why serve it any other way? Fresh corn has 280 milligrams potassium, and less than one milligram of sodium.

Canned corn? 97 milligrams potassium and 235 milligrams sodium.

Children usually love baked potatoes. Potato chips have 250 times more sodium than the same amount of baked potato. (See section on making your own chips.)

 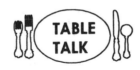

Not all children like dill pickles, but for those who do: dill pickles contain 238 times more sodium than a cucumber.

In the meat department, cured ham has 16 times more sodium than fresh pork.

And of course all children love juice. But they also enjoy fresh fruit. An average portion of fresh grapes has 158 milligrams of potassium. Compare that with the same amount of reconstituted grape juice, which only has 34 milligrams of potassium.

ADOLESCENTS
- Inappropriate eating behavior.
- Dissatisfaction with body weight.
- Discontent with appearance.
- Inappropriate approaches toward weight control.
- Fear of obesity.

Sound like portrayals of an unstable adult? *It describes an average American adolescent.*[193] The scenario worsens: Dangerous dietary restrictions — often with the mistaken intent of treating high cholesterol — cause poor growth and delayed sexual development. Similar attitudes were recently reported in elementary school students, another trend filtering down to younger and younger children.[194,195]

These consequences are serious. Decreased nutrient intake can be detected by measurements of the enzyme that activates sodium-potassium metabolism in your children's (and your!) cells. Both under- and overnutrition alter this enzyme, which is also involved with the transport of sugar and amino acids. As described, this mechanism accounts for about one-third of energy requirements. Diminished energy causes fatigue and decreases the immunological activity of the white blood cells.[196]

An extensive study on sodium-potassium blood pressure in children reported that many children have high-normal blood pressure. The good news, however, is that a reduction in sodium and/or an increase in potassium decreases the rate of rise in blood pressure during normal maturation in children and adolescents who have high-normal blood pressure.[197]

Controlled Clinical Trials, 1991

Growth retardation is associated with decreased activity of the sodium-potassium pump *without other biochemical evidence of malnutrition.* Researchers suggest that this may be a major problem in clinical pediatric practice in the United States. They conclude what you already know: The enzyme that controls the pump is sensitive to dietary intake and nutritional status.[198]

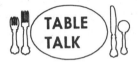

According to a Harris poll, about 80 percent of Americans are willing to pay the slight premium for organic produce. Good thing! A report from Rutgers University shows that organic tomatoes, spinach, and lettuce all have three times the potassium of the commercial varieties.

SUMMARY

There's never been a time when we have learned more about how the human body works, and what it needs to stay healthy. So far, the only thing that has contributed to healthy longevity is nutrition. We have also learned that human working parts are better off without intervention, but we have intervened. The next segment describes some simple steps you can take to compensate for this interference.

PART 3

*in which we discuss
potassium, sodium and table talk:
maintaining a healthful balance.*

POTASSIUM
IN THE KITCHEN

Okay, you're convinced. You want to get your sodium and potassium in healthful balance. After all, if you can get this dynamic duo to park and pass where and when they will function best, there's a promise of normal blood pressure, of greater energy, of longevity. But what will it take? Will you have to consume foods somewhat like a monastery recluse? Will you have to turn back the clock a thousand years? What?

If you could walk through the woods eating fruits and berries right off the vine, catch a fish here or there, eat occasional fresh-killed meat — you obviously wouldn't have to worry about that imposing sodium-potassium ratio. You would be eating as humans ate for 98.5 percent of human existence. You know that potassium is plentiful in raw, fresh, natural food, and that the sodium content in these same foods is relatively scarce. You also know your body is in favor of getting rid of potassium and will jump through hoops to hold onto its sodium.

You know that you can't live like this in the United States. You could move to the Kalahari Desert, where very little salt is consumed. Or you could join the Arctic Eskimos, Australian Aborigines, and Solomon Islanders — all of whom consume less than a gram of sodium a day (and do not develop high blood pressure). You would want to stay away from northern Japan, where the amount of salt can exceed 20 grams, or northern China, where consumption of salt is more than eight times what it is in the Amazon Jungle or in the New Guinea Highlands — or *240 times that of the Yanomama Indians of Brazil.* It is not difficult to correlate eating habits with health statistics in almost any place in the world. The entire globe becomes our laboratory, albeit an *uncontrolled* laboratory.

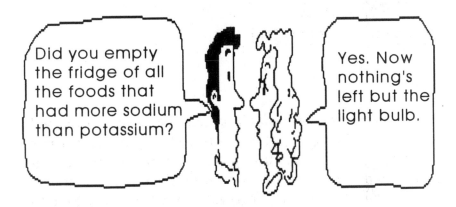

The prime approach to the modern-day problem in our western world is to seek out the freshest natural foods available, and to avoid products which have had potassium removed and sodium added. Easier said than done!

Some people actually do maintain diets close to this ideal. But this book is directed at folks like you and me who are not willing or able to devote our lives to simulating the diet of years past, however beneficial that diet may have been (even if it were ecologically and environmentally feasible). Most of us just don't have the incentive, the cooperation of other family members and friends, or the time to put it all together for such dietary goodness.

The difficulty of this kind of change is emphasized in a study of food intake, reported in *Human Nutrition; Applied Nutrition*. "Before" and "after" advice to individuals interested in eating better was scientifically validated. The results indicate that people still consume the same amount of sodium after diet changes.[1] Does this mean we are back to square one? No, because it has also been shown that a few minor nutrition changes can alter your total body and muscle potassium![2]

As herbs begin to replace salt in your kitchen, please note: Herbs should not be 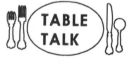 stored close to the kitchen stove. Dried herbs should be discarded and re-placed every four months. Fresh herbs are not as potent as dried,

Buy sweet butter instead of the salted variety, and add flavor by mixing these herbs into the butter: caraway, chives, garlic, parsley, or tarragon.

Instead of salt on your eggs, use basil, coriander, cress, dill, parsley, tarragon, or thyme.

Add basil, chives, dill, fennel, parsley, tarragon, or sesame seeds to fish.

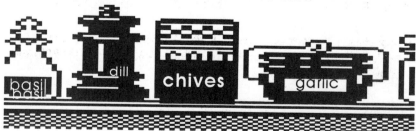

MORE POTASSIUM AND LESS SODIUM: HOW *NOT* TO DO IT

The following list of popular foods will *not* give you the sodium-potassium ratios conducive to optimal good health:

Food	Sodium	Potassium
(Milligrams per 100 grams of food)		
Apple pie	110.0	80.0
Bread, white	22.0	2.8
Cheese spreads	48.0	26.0
Cheese, American or cheddar type	30.0	2.1
Cold cuts	60.0	6.0
Corn bread	23.0	4.5
Cottage cheese	10.0	2.2
Dry cereal	4.3	3.0
Frankfurters	48.0	6.0
Green Olives	95.0	1.4
Pancakes	18.0	2.5
Peanut Butter	25.0	16.0
Peas, canned	10.0	1.2
Potato chips	42.0	11.0
Ritz Crackers	47.5	2.5
Salmon, canned	15.0	9.0
Saltines	48.0	3.0
Sauerkraut	32.0	3.5
Sponge Cake	9.0	3.0
Tuna, canned	42.0	14.0

To convert the weight of sodium to the weight of sodium chloride, multiply by 2.54. If frankfurters contain 6 mg of sodium, it contains 15.24 mg of salt as sodium chloride.

Mayo Clinic Diet Manual, 4th ed. Philadelphia, WB Saunders Co., 1971, pp 144-9.

memo:

Dr. Henry Blackburn, Department of Physiological Hygiene of the University of Minnesota, explains that high levels of sodium intake are created and maintained by the following:

- the introduction of salt to infant foods
- the heavy salting used in food processing
- the highly salted snack foods
- food traditions

Dr. Blackburn adds: *"To illustrate how salt is hidden in ordinary foods: French fries at a popular fast food restaurant contain less sodium than any of its burgers, egg dishes, milk shakes, or apple pies....Food processing in the United States drives out much of the naturally occurring potassium just as it adds salt."*[3]

One of the main reasons processed foods are so heavily salted is that salt in amounts above 3 percent result in lower microbial counts.[4] Unfortunately, salts at low concentrations can actually enhance aflatoxin production. At higher concentrations, they become inhibitory.[5] During these same procedures, potassium is leached out.[6]

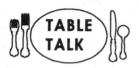

Buy your produce in a busy place, where you know there is a quick turnover — because leftovers (whether store-bought or from your own fridge) suffer nutrient losses. Don't eat foods with indeterminate ancestry. Don't eat a banana whose time was up. Too many foods available for sale have had a chance to die before purchase; many more reach their demise before they reach your table.

Salt may be used in food processing to conceal stale or rancid flavors.[7] (The use of salt for this purpose has not changed in the last few decades.) Of the ten pounds of salt ingested by each American every year, over eight pounds are already added to the food before it is purchased.[8] Salt pervades almost all processed foods, water supplies, restaurant foods, fast foods. Not only does it mask the flavor of odorous foods, but it also acts as a preservative, helps to inhibit the growth of molds and bacteria, bleaches and improves food color, and prevents discoloration.

Salt is a processing aid in peeling, sorting, and floating — useful in drying and freezing foods. As a cheap commodity, the food industry is well aware that every ounce of salt combined with foods is a saving for the manufacurer. Salt water is frequently used as a rinse for produce just prior to the canning process. Several food additives also contain sodium. It is virtually impossible to be on a salt-free diet, even if ordered by your physician.

But what about the salt you add at the dinner table? Even health enthusiasts of times long past have offered admonitions. One of my prize possessions is a book written a century and a half ago by a physician. In 1852, the good doctor said:

> The theory that additional salt in the diet is essential is miserable trash at best. Perhaps there was never a greater and more general delusion in relation to the nature, properties, and uses of common salt.
>
> Dr. R.T. Trall, M.D., Southern District of New York;
> *Hydropathic Encyclopedia*, 1852

Dr. Trall's counsel obviously has had little impact. Few listened to him then, just as similar warnings are ignored today.

The one nation that shakes more salt into its food than any other country in the world is the United States of America.

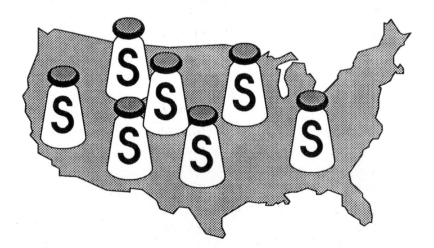

SODIUM-POTASSIUM RATIOS:
WHAT WE GET, WHAT WE NEED

Although sodium intake can be reduced, it is not always possible or practical to decrease your intake all the way down to the most desirable level — at least not without very significant personal sacrifice.

Some facts we have to live with:
1) *Facts about sodium and potassium ingested*
Understandably, numbers for an "average" sodium-potassium intake vary widely. One report claims that a typical modern North American diet includes only 1,000 milligrams of potassium and at least 2,000 milligrams of sodium per day, while some authorities indicate that a sodium-potassium ratio of 2.5 more is usual. Other accounts show a spread for the average American of 1.43 to 6.54 grams of potassium daily. Yet another source estimates that Americans consume a range of from 8 to 15 grams of sodium each and every day.[9]

2) *Facts about sodium and potassium requirements*
According to various estimates, an optimal diet includes from 1,000 to 6,000 milligrams of potassium per day, and about 250 to 1,000 milligrams of sodium per day. Official numbers from the Food and Nutrition Board are slightly different. This group states that 1,100 to 3,300 milligrams of sodium and 1,875 to 5,625 milligrams of potassium are best for "safe and adequate" intake.

Although the National Research Council has not set an RDA for potassium, it has established an "Estimated Minimum Requirement" for healthy persons: The value for adults (over the age of 10 years) is 2,000 milligrams per day, and more for the elderly.[10,11] Other researchers indicate that the absolute amount of each of these elements is not as important as the ratio between them. Some believe that dietary potassium should outweigh sodium by 3:1.[12] Others suggest that a ratio as high as ten is optimal.[13] Still others say 2:1 is fine, while some sources recommend only 1.5:1.[14]

Then there are those who point to the more natural environment of the "long ago," using this for guidance in determining what our bodies are really designed to work with. In primitive societies, the ratio of sodium to potassium in the average human diet is believed to be more like 1 to 16![15] Confusing? Whichever numbers are correct, it's safe to say we get far too much sodium and not enough potassium.

We can also differentiate between the amount of sodium and potassium that enters your mouth and how much winds up in your cells: if the ratio is well above 1:1 for the dietary (which it usually is), then the cellular ratio will be above 0.1:0.1 ratio.[16] Then there's the gender difference: the total body content of potassium in men is 140 grams; in women, 100 grams. As for sodium, it's 100 grams for men and 77 grams for women.[17] Does this mean dietary requirements for men and women should not be alike? We just don't know.

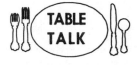

Food processing and/or refining drastically lowers potassium levels. Enriched white bread has 36 percent less potassium than whole wheat bread.[18] Be sure to check labels on whole-grain baked products. Many are mixes of depleted grains.

3) *Facts about computing your sodium and potassium intakes*
According to the Nutrition Foundation's 1990 sixth edition of *Present Knowledge in Nutrition,* even the most up-to-date state-of-the-knowledge food composition charts contain inadequate data for the potassium and/or sodium content of beverages, candies, fats and oils, cooked fish and shell fish, frozen dinners, cooked fruits, infant formulas, institutional food, processed legumes, home-prepared mixed dishes, restaurant food, many snack foods, and cooked vegetables.[19] So even if you did walk

through the supermarket with a computer and a book of charts, your computations cannot be accurate.

Here's one example: Banana- and apricot-containing baby foods (reconstituted from concentrate) were checked for official values for potassium. The results were far less than the postings in the United States Department of Agriculture Handbook No. 8-9.[20]

In testing your body chemistry for potassium deficiency, you may have a loss of potassium in brain tissue, but your blood levels could appear to be normal.[21] Similarly, the amount of potassium in your blood serum is usually different from the amount of potassium in your red blood cells.[22]

4) *Facts about minor potassium deficiencies*
Minor shortages of potassium can bring on vague weakness, impairment of neuromuscular function, poor reflexes and mental confusion. The point is that it doesn't take major inadequacies to cause a problem.

5) *Facts about potassium absorption*
Although potassium may be present in your orange juice, cofactors necessary for its assimilation may be missing. The *American Dietetic Association* reported on the nutrient content and labeling of several processed Florida citrus juice products. Samples (frozen concentrated orange juice, orange juice from concentrate, pasteurized orange juice, grapefruit juice, and grapefruit juice from concentrate) were surveyed regularly for a two-year period *at the time of packing*. They were assayed for various nutrients. Potassium remained intact in what the researchers believed to be "significant" quantities. The fate of other nutrients — including those required as cofactors for potassium absorption — was not as successful.

To be claimed on a label, a nutrient must occur at a minimum level of 2 percent of the U.S. RDA per serving, according to Food and Drug Administration regulations. So if a product contains only 1.2 milligrams of vitamin C per serving, the label could read, "CONTAINS VITAMIN C". RDA requirements are deemed by many researchers to be far too low in any case. Two percent of "already low" is, as one researcher described it, "obscene."

Despite the low standard, neither zinc nor iron was found in the Florida citrus products tested at this RDA minimum level of 2 percent; only a very small percentage of B vitamins was evident; and small (but claimable) levels of magnesium, calcium, copper, and phosphorus were found. Since potassium works synergistically with other nutrients, how useful is the potassium in your processed orange juice? Your guess is as good as any.[23] (B_6, for example, is necessary for efficient potassium absorption. And magnesium is a *must* for driving potassium into the cells.)

Note that the testing was done at the same time as packing. Further losses are incurred with storage and exposure to variations in temperature.

Salads and salad dressings can be spruced up with basil, chives, cress, dill, garlic, marjoram, oregano, parsley, savory, and/or tarragon. Flavor your homemade soups with basil, bay leaf, chives, dill, oregano, parsley, tarragon, capsicum, and curry powder for "hot" soup. Caveat: Restaurant and canned soups are heavily salted.

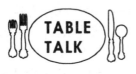

MORE POTASSIUM AND LESS SODIUM: HOW TO DO IT

It appears that we are left with one inescapable conclusion: The ratio of sodium to potassium is likely to be far too high. Even if you do get "enough" potassium to meet the accepted minimum, critical cofactors may be missing. So if you want to increase your potassium intake, the questions remaining are: how and how much?

Food is your best source for potassium, as it is for nearly all nutrients. By now you are aware that in a relatively natural, unmolested form, foods almost always contain a lot less sodium than potassium. In most plants the ratio is typically about 1:20. In animals (and very healthy humans), a ratio of 1:3 is more common.

If you are in charge of preparing your own meals, you can dramatically increase the amount of potassium in your food and decrease salt intake by adopting some of the suggestions in the Table Talk hints posted throughout this section.

Nearly all of the best sources of potassium are raw fruits, raw or minimally-cooked vegetables, and nuts (cracked open as you eat them to avoid rancidity), with a few examples of fresh fish and high quality cuts of meat. But now let's confront reality. If you're like most North Americans, your diet is probably something you would rather not discuss in public — at least not without excuses and apologies. You may go for days and never consume these foods in their fresh and natural form. I'll spare you the standard rant against overprocessed convenience foods. Note the chart earlier in this chapter. It is obvious that these foods can affect your sodium-potassium ratio if they dominate your diet. Study the list again, and look at the following chart of high-potassium foods. Think about what you eat in a typical day.

High Potassium Foods
per 100 grams edible portion

Dulse	8060
Kelp	5273
Irishmoss	2844
Pistachio nuts	972
Dehydrated prunes	940
Sunflower seeds	920
Dried lentils	790
Raisins	763
Parsley	727
Dried prunes	694
Cress	606
Avocado	604
Yams	600
Beet greens	570
Water chestnuts	500
Spinach	470
Millet	430
Potato with skin	407
Banana	370
Carrots	341

These figures are based on 100 grams, or the amount equal to the size of your fist — a fairly good-sized portion.

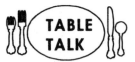

When ordering in the Chinese restaurant, ask for more water chestnuts. (And, for reasons defined in *New Facts About Fiber*, you should also be requesting brown rice.)

A few pointers:

➤Commercially dried fruits are frequently laced with sulphur dioxide, an antibrowning preservative. Sulphured fruits are brighter, plumper, moister, and "fresher" looking.[24] In large doses, sulfites can cause gastric irritation, colic, and diarrhea. In any dose, they may cause serious circulatory disturbances to the sensitive, including asthmatics. Sulfites also destroy nutrients. (See section later in this chapter on home dehydration.)

➤Kelp, even though it has a very high sodium content, can still boast even more potassium! *Natural, intact foods, even if high in sodium, contain more potassium.*

➤The following are potassium antagonists — substances which deplete your much-needed potassium:

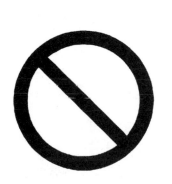

alcohol
antibiotics[25]
caffeine
diarrhea
diuretics
excessive sweating
high cholesterol levels
hormone products:
    cortisone, aldosterone
inflammation relievers: colchicine
laxatives
salt
stress
sugar

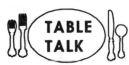

A tablespoon of horseradish contains 17 milligrams of sodium, but **TABLE TALK** offers 52 milligrams of potassium. Horseradish provides taste and texture. Good for chicken, meats, fish.

The task of potassium-enhancement with food becomes fairly effortless once you decide you can add a few veggies to your daily routine. In fact, it's much easier than obtaining most vitamins or other essential nutrients in the same manner, because potassium, since it is an element, is not going to break down as easily, especially when cooked properly at low temperatures. Nor will it oxidize and turn rancid with age or improper treatment.

Potassium is present in large quantities in such a wide variety of foods that there's little excuse for not finding a good source that you like. If you don't like bananas, how about potatoes (with the skin). If you don't want a potato, try a slice of avocado.

YOUR CHOICE!

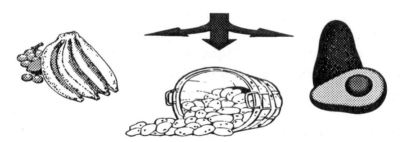

Or you might be more interested in sunflower seeds. For several decades I have recommended sunflower seeds as an ideal snack for many reasons. Here's one more argument to add to the list: Sunflower seeds offer 920 milligrams of potassium per 100 grams (about a quarter of a pound), among the highest potassium values for foods analyzed in the United States Department of Agriculture Handbook No. 8. Bananas and oranges, contain respectively only 370 milligrams and 200 milligrams per 100 grams.[26]

To increase the nutrient value of sunflower seeds, and to offset any 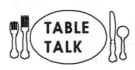 rancidity present if you purchase your seeds already shelled, soak seeds overnight in water about an inch above the level of the seeds (that is, somewhat more than enough to cover). Drain in the morning and spread out on a plate. Rinse (in a strainer) at night. Spread again. The next morning, add to salads or munch. Here's the procedure:

- Soak overnight.
- Rinse in morning. Spread out to drain.
- Rinse at night. Spread out to drain.
- Use next day. Refrigerate if not consumed early in day.

One of the problems with some potassium-rich foods is that they can be very sweet. (This does not refer to added sugar — we're limiting our discussion to foods that have not been tampered with.) The ubiquitous banana, one of the most potent sources of dietary potassium, also comes with a high dose of fruit sugar. A carrot or a celery stick makes a better potassium snack for those with blood sugar (too high or too low) or weight problems.

Many North Americans are hypoglycemic to some extent, suffering from low blood sugar, caused by the bodies' inability to fully cope with the incredibly unnatural onslaught of sweetened foods in the western diet. If sugar is a concern, the list of acceptable potassium-bearing foods narrows a little. For others, the natural sugar content in most foods will not be a problem.

Even though eating a potassium-rich diet *should* be easy, we know that there are situations when it might not be. If you're rushed for breakfast (or often have to skip it), have a quick lunch (perhaps in the company cafeteria), or eat dinner out (as often as in), your options may be very limited. Countervailing trends in the use of convenience foods increase the difficulty for all of us to lower sodium intake.

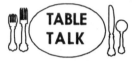

(For diabetics and hypoglycemics) When eating sweet potassium foods, eat them with fiber. Fiber helps to flatten (or normalize) your *glycemic, or blood sugar,* response. (Example: When I eat a banana, I slice it into whole grain cereal, eat a handful of mung and/or lentil sprouts, munch a fiber bar, or mix up a fiber drink.)

To ascertain the cooking losses of minerals, including potassium, foods were analyzed before and after cooking, and the following results were obtained, as reported in the *Journal of Nutritional Science and Vitaminology*:

(1) Mineral contents of cooked foods in mass cooking were about 60 to 70 percent of those in raw or uncooked foods.

(2) Cooking losses of minerals were particularly high in vegetables.

(3) Among various cooking methods, losses were largest in squeezing after boiling and in soaking in water after thin-slicing, followed by parching, frying and stewing.

(4) Cooking losses in meals cooked at home brought about similar results as those by the mass-cooking procedures.

(5) The measures to prevent cooking loss are
   • eating the boiled food with the soup
   • avoidance of too much boiling
   • using a cooking method causing less mineral
     loss (stewing, stir-frying, or parching).[28]

Don't overcook foods to the point that cell walls and membranes are 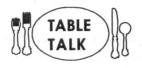 destroyed, thereby allowing the potassium-rich liquid within the cells to be physically altered or washed away with the cooking water. Potatoes, for example, lose potassium when they are boiled.[27] When you have a choice, steam, rather than boil.

I'd rather die than stop eating junk foods.

Careful. You may get your wish.

NO SALT INSURANCE

SALT SUBSTITUTES

Even though you know that adding table salt (sodium chloride) to food for flavor is a very destructive habit, you may not be sufficiently motivated to change this habit. I understand; I have habits, too. A wise man is reported to have said, *"Person would sooner give up spouse than dietary habits."* Fortunately, there are alternatives in the form of salt substitutes. But, caveat emptor:

Thirteen commercially available salt-substitute products were analyzed for content. Here are the results, as reported in the *Journal of the American Dietetic Association*:

- sodium values ranged from 2 milligrams to 2,180 milligrams per teaspoon
- sodium-potassium ratios were as low as 0.07 but as high as 2,460 per teaspoon
- calcium and magnesium levels in most seasonings were modest
- kelp-based seasonings provided about 50 milligrams of calcium and 35 of magnesium per teaspoon[29]

Many of the commercial salt substitutes, or "light" salt products simply replace potassium chloride for some of the sodium chloride of table salt. Although this does introduce some needed potassium, the chloride form happily aids in the reabsorption of sodium in your kidneys, thereby compromising the effectiveness of this type of salt substitute.[30] The products that use potassium citrate or other combinations of potassium are preferred.

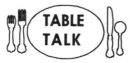

TABLE TALK

Most herbs should be added in moderation during the last stages of cooking. If cooked too long, they may give a bitter taste to foods.

SALT ALTERNATIVES

If used excessively, salt substitutes containing potassium may help induce a dangerous level of potassium.[31] So your best bet is to go for salt *alternatives*. Although not endowed with the taste of ordinary salt, these products are very rich in natural potassium and a host of other important minerals.

Salt alternatives are not really salt substitutes because they don't pretend to emulate the taste, tang, or characteristic of salt. They offer different flavors that stand on their own — taking your mind off the desire for salt. Among salt alternatives:

> onion, garlic, horseradish (watch out — some brands contain lots of salt), dry mustard, chili, tabasco, curry, lemon juice, oregano, pepper, Worcestershire sauce, and sage.

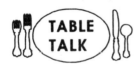

For the die-hards who salt before they taste, the following herbs have a salty flavor: summer savory, lovage, and celery. Or, while in transition, you could replace the contents of the salt shaker with this composite: 1 tablespoon of ground coarse salt (coarse salt has more flavor than the overprocessed free-flowing variety, so you use less), ¼ tablepoon each of ground black peppercorns, ground coriander seeds, ground bay leaves, and dried basil. Slowly reduce the salt content and increase other condiments.

And you thought life without table salt would be dull!

POTASSIUM SUPPLEMENTATION

Nutrients are only useful when they go where you want them to go — when they are bioavailable at the cellular level. In other words, they have to cross your cell membranes. As explained, absorption and transportation of minerals involve complex biochemical systems.

Potassium supplementation may be a practical consideration. Such supplements fall into three categories: solid (pills), liquid (swallowed by the spoonful) and salt substitutes (described above). Liquid supplements are always more efficiently and more quickly assimilated, having the same benefits as sublingual preparations (the kind you place under your tongue for quick absorption). A chemist who develops nutrient formulas said to me, "After extensive study, I believe that liquid supplements are better in today's world because we're so glued up from the pizzas and gluten. Our livers are not detoxifying as well as they should any longer."

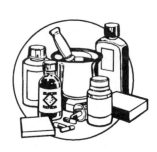

The consequences of taking supplements are very different from those resulting from drugs. You don't usually get an instant boost with the more natural ingredients — effects are usually somewhat slower (but longer lasting when they do kick in). The advantage? No side effects, and, unlike drugs, the action doesn't continue if not needed.

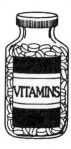

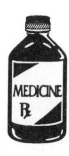

WHICH POTASSIUM SUPPLEMENT?

Bioavailability of a nutrient is dependent on the chemical form as well as the concentration of other dietary constituents such as fiber, phytate, carbohydrates, macrominerals, and vitamins in the diet.[31] Like all other nutrients that we attempt to spoon-feed, the form of potassium influences just how efficiently it will be handled in your body. Note the following:

• Potassium glycerophosphate

Potassium glycerophosphate is produced by an involved and unique process which takes four or five days in the making. Once you swallow it, however, it is assimilated quickly and is known for its excellent quality and high efficiency. Because this form of potassium is already bonded, difficulties that may beset other forms of potassium are nonexistent. Potassium glycerophosphate penetrates cell walls easily through a mechanical, rather than an electrical, process. This spares energy!

You would have to consume many dozens of tablets to glean the advantages of a dose of liquid potassium glycerophosphate.

• Potassium citrate

Potassium citrate is well-tolerated and readily absorbed. It is useful therapeutically because it can often restore normal urinary citrate. Citrate is important because it retards the crystallization of stone-forming calcium salts. But its level in urine is low as a result of dietary aberrations, *including sodium excess* and elevated intake of animal proteins.[33] Potassium citrate also reduces urinary calcium excretion, thereby improving calcium balance.[34]

• Potassium/magnesium aspartate

Aspartates are minerals bound to the salt of aspartic acid. The potassium and magnesium ions, when transported to the inner layer of the outer cell membrane, activate energy-rich phosphates, which in turn activate energy-producing enzymes.

• Potassium chloride

Potassium chloride is found in salt substitutes, and in some supplements. As mentioned earlier, the chloride that remains when the potassium is utilized may contribute to the retention of additional sodium, thereby defeating the purpose of the potassium supplementation. High levels, which would be necessary for supplementation, can cause gastrointestinal discomfort.[35,36] Potassium chloride also interferes with vitamin B_{12} absorption. The depletion of one nutrient affects the requirement for another, so it may be a round-robin of no-good effects.[37]

It isn't often that we read about "natural" therapies in traditional medical journals. The *American Journal of Hypertension* reports that a potassium preparation is an effective means of decreasing sodium and increasing potassium intake, and may be used for antihypertensive treatment in mild hypertension.[38] A German medical journal reported that potassium levels (along with magnesium) should be controlled and corrected by ingestion of electrolyte preparations for cardiac health.[39]

Try chopped chervil leaves for cream soups; dill for consommé or sliced tomatoes; chives 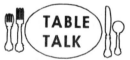 and/or chervil for baked potatoes; mint for potatoes or peas; thyme for turkey; savory for deviled eggs.

And here's a helpful herb/vegetable list:

squash ➤ basil
onions ➤ bay leaf
carrots ➤ dill
peas ➤ marjoram
mushrooms ➤ oregano
green beans ➤rosemary
onions ➤ saffron
lentils ➤ savory
celery ➤ tarragon
beets ➤ thyme

WHEN AND HOW TO TAKE YOUR SUPPLEMENT

Nutrients interact, so it's a good idea to take your supplements with meals. One study shows there is no significant difference when potassium citrate is given with or between meals.[40]

The old cliché that *you are what you eat* has long since dissolved into *you are what you absorb.* It was my friend Larry Jordan, to whom this book is dedicated, who set me on the trail of potassium investigation. My sleuthing confirmed that for an element like potassium to be effective, it must be *properly* absorbed, which means it should be accompanied by other food-type constituents — the more natural, the better. For me this means taking a supplement with these requirements:

- The potassium must be in its best Sunday dress (for example, something like potassium glycerophosphate or potassium citrate rather than potassium chloride).

- The supplement should contain no more potassium than you might find in about two bananas, since I don't want to be on potassium overload.

- The supplement has to be accompanied by a mixture of food-type substances to help insure normal metabolism. Potassium, like all nutrients, requires *other* nutrients in order to do its job properly.
  (a) The hormonal control of potassium is mediated through the adrenal cortex hormones and hormones of the anterior pituitary gland.[41]
  (b) Retention of potassium is facilitated and ensured by magnesium.[42,43] The heart muscle cannot hold onto potassium in the absence of magnesium.[44] *Magnesium is necessary for the sodium-potassium pump.*[45]
  (c) Vitamin B_6 offers neighborly assistance to potassium metabolism, also helping to secure the adequacy of potassium.[46]

So I take my potassium in a brew of nutrient-dense products which offer a range of cofactor constituents. We're past the point of using a single whole plant all by itself in supplemental form. Whole plant *mixtures* or fractions of plant combinations provide activity not achieved in other ways. The variety helps to assure the presence of nutrients necessary for potassium assimilation.

A significant lesson we've learned in nutrition in the past few years is that one nutrient is interdependent on another, and another, and yet another. The more different foods you eat, the higher the chance of obtaining the nutrients you require. By the same token, a supplement could have a variety of special ingredients.

Herbs in supplements may also act as a preservative if they are present in high enough quantity, and if they are generally adaptogenic. Since their active constituents are more or less held in abeyance if your body doesn't require them, most herbs are safe in small quantities.

Fresh herbs are preferable when available. Rule of thumb is to use twice the amount of fresh herbs as you would 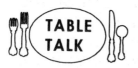 dried. Dried herbs have a stronger, more concentrated flavor.

TABLE TALK

VALIDATING POTASSIUM SUPPLEMENTATION

Can't we just make a majestic effort to reduce sodium intake and let it go at that? The answer is *no*. An article in *Hypertension* addresses general and specific aspects of dietary sodium interventions from the perspective of *behavioral* change which requires relearning a range of habits. These habits are involved in day-to-day eating situations in the context of a diverse and complex food supply and in consideration of numerous factors — other than health concerns — which influence habitual eating patterns. Obstacles to dietary sodium reduction relate to the wide distribution of sodium in foods, strong cultural values about the place of salt in the diet and difficulty in assessing success in sodium reduction.

A review of reports of sodium interventions suggest that state-of-the-art behavioral change strategies can be effective in achieving reductions in sodium intake to around 3,000 milligrams a day but that this level is achieved only with highly motivated individuals, and then only when a high level of intervention is provided.

So, in regard to sodium reduction in the general population, either the goal has to be modest or the food supply will have to change.[47] Modest goals do not make for optimum health, and we all know the food supply is not about to change. In fact, most of the salt is in commercially prepared foods, and their consumption, according to Mark Hegsted, renowned nutritionist reporting in *Hypertension*, will increase in the future.[48]

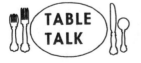

Restaurant tip: Order a side dish of vegetables instead of the menu's appetizers when dining in an elegant restaurant. A really good establishment will be happy to accommodate. Ask that all sauces be placed on the side. Take nothing for granted.

To validate the use of potassium supplementation, note the following studies:

➤*Hypertension*, Nov 1991: Dietary potassium supplementation reduces pressure in hypertension.[49]

➤*Annals of Internal Medicine*, Nov 1991: Increasing dietary potassium diminishes the need for antihypertensive medication.[50]

➤*Journal of Urology*, Sep 1991: Potassium citrate decreases urinary saturation of calcium oxalate and uric acid.[51]

➤*The Nutrition Report*, Aug 1991: Potassium supplementation:
  • lowers blood pressure in hypertensive individuals
  • reduces medication requirements
  • protects against effects of salt on arterial pressure[52]

➤*Postgraduate Medicine* Jul 1991: Potassium supplementation lowers blood pressure.[53]

➤*Versicherungsmedizin*, Jun 1991: Low-calorie diets of poor nutritional value are risky. Ingestion of electrolyte preparations containing potassium can help to mitigate deleterious effects.[54]

➤*Journal of Hypertension*, May 1991: Oral potassium supplements significantly lower blood pressure. The magnitude of the blood-pressure lowering effect is greater in patients with high blood pressure and appears to be more pronounced the longer the duration of the supplementation.[55]

➤*Journal of the American College of Nutrition*, Apr 1991: Increased potassium exerts a protective effect among elderly men against hypertension when sodium exposure is relatively high.[56]

➤*Journal of Human Hypertension*, Apr 1991: Potassium supplementation lowers blood pressure.[57]

➤*Journal of Cardiovascular Pharmacology*, Feb 1991: Results support the notion that potassium supplementation may be an effective therapeutic approach to mildly hypertensive blacks.[58]

➤*Journal of Hypertension*, Feb 1991: Potassium supplementation lowers blood pressure in test animals.[59]

➤*American Journal of Physiology*, Jan 1991: Potassium supplementation tended to decrease sodium "space" in hypertensive test animals.[60]

➤*Nutrition and Cancer*, 1990: Supplemental potassium helps to partially prevent tumors in test animals, reducing the tumor incidence from 40 to 5 percent. Additional good news is that the level of potassium supplements used cause no toxic effects.[61]

➤*Age and Aging*, 1990: After double-blind crossover trials, the researchers conclude that potassium therapy is a safe therapy.[62]

➤*Journal of the Formosan Medical Association*, Dec 1990: Clinical symptoms of tenderness and weakness of the extremity muscles improved after administration of a few macronutrients, including potassium.[63]

➤*Schwizerische Rundschau fur Medizin Praxis*, Sep 1990: Increased administration of potassium is among the suggestions for reducing hypertension as an alternative to drugs in mild hypertension.[64]

➤*Drugs*, Jul 1990: Thiazide diuretics cause impaired glucose tolerance in diabetics, but with potassium supplementation the adverse effect is lessened.[65]

➤*Gesamte Innere Medizin und Ihre Grenzgebiete,* Jun 1990 :According to German medical studies, blood pressure reduction with the use of omega-3 fatty acids can be improved by an additional increase in potassium intake.[66]

➤*American Journal of Cardiology,* Mar 1990: Potassium deficiency may be as powerful a determinant of cardiovascular morbidity and mortality as sodium excess. In patients with chronic heart failure, potassium can modify both the mechanical and electrical properties of the heart, it can exert diuretic effects, and it can reduce the frequency and complexity of potentially lethal ventricular tachyarrhythmias. Given this central role, the effects can be enhanced or diminished by potassium homeostasis.[67]

Changes in potassium levels clearly have significance:
   •They affect the membrane potential of vascular smooth muscle cells.
   •They influence the levels and activity of hormones affecting blood pressure.
   •They influence the levels and activity of intracellular messengers involved in vasoconstriction.
   •They alter the body's handling of sodium.

The net result is that, perhaps of these phenomena, chronic supplementation of dietary potassium is associated with improved health.[68]

Hospital Practice (Office Edition), 1988

➤*American Journal of Cardiology*, 1990: An increased intake of potassium (*without a change in dietary sodium*) can reduce blood pressure, may suppress the activity of the sympathetic nervous and renin-angiotensin systems, and can prevent development of vascular injury; conversely, potassium depletion has been associated with an increase in stroke and sudden death.[69]

➤*Advances in Experimental Medicine and Biology*, 1989: Potassium supplements improve the body's retention of copper.[70]

➤*Kidney International*, Feb 1989: Potassium bicarbonate supplementation promotes more positive calcium balances.[71]

➤*Hospital Practice* (Office Edition), Dec 1988: Potassium repletion even for mildly depressed levels is vitally important. Indications are emerging demonstrating that potassium supplementation may be valuable in preventing renal damage and stroke, quite apart from any effect on hypertension itself.[72]

➤*The Paleolithic Prescription*, 1988: Excessive sodium and minimal potassium lead the way to hypertension. Even in animals with well-established hypertension, high-potassium diets prolonged the average length of life. Potassium intake may ultimately be part of the solution.[73]

➤*Journal of Clinical Endocrinology Metabolism*, 1986: Potassium citrate may benefit people who tend to form kidney stones because citrate augments the inhibitor activity against calcium oxalate crystallization.[74]

➤*Hypertension*, 1985: Adding potassium to the normal chow reduced the mortality from 83 percent to 2 percent in stroke-prone hypertensive test animals. The added potassium seemed to prevent lesions in the cerebral arteries and deaths even when blood-pressure lowering was eliminated as a factor. The potassium offered protection against brain hemorrhage.[75]

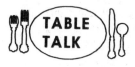

TABLE TALK Restaurant tip:Order a variety of vegetables, quickly stir-fried and seasoned with garlic or ginger (or both) when in an Asian restaurant. Don't be embarrassed to ask that the salt (and the MSG) be omitted.

➤*Journal of Urology*, 1985: During the three years prior to treatment, calcium stone-forming patients formed an average of 39 to 40 stones each. Treatment with oral potassium citrate over a thirty-four-month period resulted in complete inhibition of new stone formation in all patients.[76]

➤*Annals of Internal Medicine*, 1986: Potassium citrate therapy over a two-year period resulted in an 86 percent reduction in stone formation rate.[77]

➤*European Journal of Clinical Investigation*, 1984: Potassium supplementation accompanying a diet is associated with better insulin and glucose utilization.[78]

➤*Lancet*, 1982: Twenty healthy males received either increased potassium or a placebo (a product that looks like the real thing, but has no value) while on a normal sodium unrestricted diet. A significantly greater proportion had lower blood pressure on the potassium than on the placebo.[79]

Many of the studies cited were double-blind, crossover, randomized trials — protocols that should satisfy the most exacting scrutiny of scientific critics.

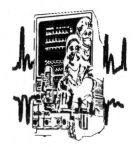

Since I've been eating lots of vegetables and taking my supplements, I don't get sick any more.

My doctor is suing me for alienation of infections.

I can hear it now, the critics saying, "Eat a balanced diet and you don't *need* supplementation!" If only that were true! It is my hope that reading this and other books on the subject inspires you to decrease salt, and increase the vegetables on your dinner plate. Even if you are eating in such exemplary style, you are still not home-free. Note this commentary by Dr. Jesse A. Stoff:

Many nutrients found in decreased amounts in synthetically fertilized vegetables are now being revealed as essential to the intracellular metabolism in fighting off a variety of disorders and diseases. Thus eating "good" foods alone will not ensure adequate levels of vitamins and minerals any more. Certain nutritional supplements can not only increase the supply of essential nutrients, but also have specific therapeutic effects.[80]

A suggestion for those who dine out frequently is to choose ethnic 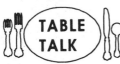 cuisine (Chinese, Thai, or Indian, for example). These generally offer a variety of healthful menu selections, with a broader choice of fresh vegetables.

memo:

A SURVEY IN THE ROLE OF NUTRITION

PROTECTIVE FACTORS IN THE
PREVENTION OF
HIGH CHOLESTEROL AND
HEART DISEASE:
n-3 and n-6 polyunsaturated
fatty acids; oleic acid, plant
sterols, plant lecithins, fiber
components, plant proteins
(e.g. soybeans), vitamin C,
vitamin E, **potassium**, calcium,
chromium, magnesium, and
selenium.

RISK FACTORS FOR
HIGH CHOLESTEROL AND
HEART DISEASE:
sucrose, **sodium**, alcohol,
excessive vitamin D, alcohol.

POSSIBLE DANGERS OF
POTASSIUM SUPPLEMENTATION

Although your body does a good job of getting rid of excess potassium through adaptation (kidney elimination is normally enhanced in the presence of excess),[81] there are some cautions. Please don't take any old potassium supplement. Potassium supplementation is not risk-free. Adults taking diuretics, for example, should proceed with caution. As already noted, most diuretics cause a potassium deficiency. But some work in a way that *preserves* potassium, so there should be no deficit to make up beyond the usual dietary needs. Again, the safe side is to take a low-dose potassium supplement (again: a supplement with no more potassium than the amount found in two bananas).

The sodium-potassium control systems of infants, and possibly children, are many times more fragile than those of adults. Do not even think about giving potassium supplements to infants or very young children unless such a supplement is recommended by your doctor, and you are certain that the potassium content is not excessively high.

 I cannot overemphasize the fact that such a supplement should be taken concomitantly with natural-type ingredients or, better still, such ingredients should be blended with your potassium.

Solid forms of potassium supplements pose a relatively minor risk to adults in a completely different way. If the capsule remains stationary for a long period of time while it dissolves, there is some risk of intestinal ulcers.[82]

WHAT OTHER THINGS SHOULD YOU DO?

Potassium is only one small part of good nutrition. The following statement appears in the 1991 *Annual Review of Medicine*:

> It is important to recognize that nutrients are not ingested in isolation, but as interactive constituents of a total diet. Moreover, failure to appreciate the interactive influences may result in other than the desired effect.[83]

TWO OTHER TRACE ELEMENTS OF SIGNIFICANCE
Magnesium

Magnesium has a critically important roles in human nutrition. It is one of the factors that regulates the transport of ions across the cell membrane.[84] Your reserve to combat magnesium depletion is not designed to protect the *extracellular* magnesium pool or certain critical organs. A continuous optimal intake of magnesium is needed for good nutrition and health. But while magnesium is the most directly related to potassium due to its role in muscle and nerve mechanisms, other minerals are also important.

Chromium

Chromium is another mineral of importance. Chromium is found in required amounts in most young children, but is not detected at all in 15 to 23 percent of Americans over the age of fifty. Yet 98.5 percent of most non-Americans in that age category can boast its presence in sufficient amounts. Short supplies subject almost everyone to many problems, both subtle and serious. Chromium functions in a special niacin-bound organic complex called *glucose tolerance factor* (GTF), which regulates carbohydrate, fat, and protein metabolism in the production of energy and in cholesterol management.

EXERCISE

This section is only for those of you who do not exercise. That probably means most of you, because only a minority of adults in our affluent society engages in appropriate regular physical activity.

If high blood pressure is your primary concern — and even if it isn't — exercise is universally recognized as an effective way to improve the condition of your arteries. *Strenuous short-term exercise has a favorable outcome on potassium status.*[85] The easiest way to get such exercise is to walk fast for about 20 minutes, at least 3 times a week.

In a study done with people aged 48-59 years, those who engaged in regular exercise for thirty days, showed better potassium, sodium and chloride metabolism and a normalization of hormone levels — in contrast to other groups of subjects not exercising.[86]

Did you know that you get the same benefit out of thirty minutes of brisk walking as you get from twenty minutes of running? Long periods of vigorous walking do more to reduce fat than brief sessions of jogging. Aerobic exercises are those that make your heart accelerate for a sustained period of time, causing a need for more air (oxygen). So an aerobic exercise is go-go-go, not stop-and-go. Aerobic *walking* is best.

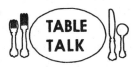

Taking a substantial dose of vitamin C before exercising improves coronary reserve and reduces risk. Since vitamin C deficiency can sabotage airway response to exercise, treatment with vitamin C ahead of time may prevent these problems.[87]

ADAPTOGENS

What's an adaptogen? A substance that seems to have no specific function — until it is needed, that is, it *adapts* to your needs. Adaptogens have positive actions against a wide range of serious conditions. They are almost always user-friendly and are classified as nontoxic. They are known to enhance your ability to cope with any stress — physical, emotional, or chemical.

Adaptogens differ from drugs in several ways. No prescriptions are necessary. No high-tech equipment, needles, syringes, or professional expertise is required for administration. They are less costly than most drugs. They are not-habit forming. A drug continues to work even after a state of normalcy is achieved. An adaptogen regulates, and is held in abeyance when the challenge ceases to exist.

Pollen

Pollen is the male seed of flowers, and, like any seed, it contains across-the-board nutrients. Each pollen grain has from one million to five million pollen spores, all capable of reproducing the species. Bee pollen has been touted as a "perfect" food.

This golden dust is comprised of thousands of enzymes and coenzymes — *many times more than in any other food.* An enzyme is a kind of catalyst: the hammer that drives the nail, a substance that facilitates or promotes a biological reaction. Enzymes can only be processed by a living organism.

Pollen does not necessarily have to be processed by the bees. One excellent product uses pollen directly from the flower. This enables the pollen to be harvested mechanically under controlled conditions, offering a supplement of quality and distinction. Non-chemical processes parallel those performed naturally by bees, with the advantage of select-flower use and reduced variations.

Acidophilus

What? Add more bacteria to your gut? Yes, the good-guy variety, to crowd out bacteria of direputable lineage. You can resist enemy invasion by entrenching your normal flora with healthful sentries. The easiest way to provide a settlement of proper bacteria is with acidophilus. A good acidophilus supplement loads a few billion acidophilus organisms per gram. The acidophilus bacteria set up housekeeping in your intestine, creating an ecological system that helps to absorb nutrients and create new ones.

Acidophilus is available in a milk base, or vegetarian-grown. A similar helpful bacterium (*lactobacillus bulgaricus*, perhaps a second cousin once removed) is found in *viable* yogurt. (Note the emphasis on *viable*; not all supermarket yogurts are "live." Natural food store proprietors can direct you to the "live" yogurt.)

Your great-grandmother produced another equally beneficial strain by "clabbering," or souring, milk in her kitchen. Nearly every society consumes a fermented or cultured food product of one type or another because empirical observation shows that the addition of these foods is associated with good health. According to conclusions reached at an international medical symposium in Sweden, such products are of extreme importancc in the nutrition of people everywhere. Fermentation is one of the most important functions of the colonic flora.

There are more living entities in your flora than there are cells in your whole body. Acidophilus contributes favorably to your microflora, performing a wide variety of important functions in nutrition, immunology, and metabolism in general.

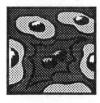 Long ago, the process was initiated by organisms present in raw foods, in the air, or on utensils. Today we use specific starter cultures and precise conditions of time and temperature, insuring superior products and microbial safety.

Garlic

Garlic! A favorite adaptogen. Research validates that garlic can influence the course of a host of modern ailments, including heart disease, several types of cancer and cell damage caused by pollutants, radiation and aging.

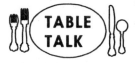 Deodorized forms of garlic may work as well as pure, unadulterated fresh garlic.

Probably the most important constituent of garlic is a chemical called allicin, the sulphurous and smelly substance that also seems to give garlic most of its outstanding medicinal qualities. Allicin is a natural antibiotic — it has even been compared favorably with penicillin for the treatment of certain classes of infections. But allicin in its active form is relatively scarce in fresh garlic. Its precursor, alliin, must be converted to allicin by the enzyme allinase. These two substance are found on opposite sides of cell walls, however, and do not mix until the garlic is either digested or physically altered — explaining why the garlic smell becomes so strong when garlic is crushed.

Trace nutrients such as selenium and germanium are relatively abundant in garlic. (Selenium is a powerful antioxidant; germanium is thought to have tremendous importance for immune functions.) And guess what other mineral is found in quantity in garlic? *Potassium* — 529 milligrams in 100 grams of garlic!

In addition, certain groupings of sulfur and oxygen in garlic oil have recently been shown to have bactericidal properties.

My recommendation to eat lots of garlic is usually easy advice to follow. If you don't like garlic (or if it doesn't like you), there are excellent garlic-based supplements available, the so-called "sociable" variety. A quality preparation is comprised of garlic that has gone through a long-term natural cold-aging process. The alliin is converted to beneficial sulfur compounds, and the final product is odorless. The antimicrobial mechanisms of garlic supplements have explained some of its effects. One study shows how garlic supplements induced increased natural killer cell activity. And test animals given this elixir have been able to resist the flu! The successful merging of traditional wisdom with high technology is something to be respected.

Dr. James Duke, an economic botanist for the Department of Agriculture who is assisting the National Cancer Institute as a researcher, began to study the link between garlic and cancer after noting the amounts of garlic eaten in certain provinces of China and the low incidence of cancer there.

We have been learning a lot about longevity from the Japanese, who have the longest life expectancy in the world. The first extractions of the essence of garlic came to us from Japan. I had an opportunity to visit garlic fields in Hiroshima, and to witness first-hand the organic growing conditions. The active elements of garlic cloves are extracted over a twenty-month period before thay are concentrated and aged in outdoor tanks. (In true Japanese fashion, the tanks were surrounded by formal gardens.)

I also saw garlic growing in a remote area of Japan, selected for its lack of pollution. I stood at the edge of a field, not too far from Siberia, and contemplated how fortunate Americans are to have such products available — as though the thousands of distant miles between the fields, the labs, and our kitchen tables were nonexistent.

I went through many rooms of garlic laboratories, witnessing first-hand the 250 tests conducted to get from raw garlic to finished product, and to observe the involvement in commitment to research and development. A fascinating experience, which only confirmed my belief in this wonderful product.

Herbs

The cornucopia of nutrients present in herbs (which make some of them sound like snake oil) is not uncommon to adaptogenic substances. Many wonderful herbs grace the marketplace. Suffice it to say that herbs such as chamomile, alfalfa, sarsaparilla root, passion flower, dandelion root, and so on, have stood the test of time as healing substances. We find references to herbs in use as early as 2500 B.C. Clay tablets record the attributes of some two hundred and fifty herbs.

In addition to their express use as healing aids and in the cosmetic industry, their use in the kitchen is highly recommended. Here are a few favorite recipes.

Tarragon Vinegar Salad Dressing

Combine ¼ teaspoon pepper; ¼ teaspoon dry mustard; 1 teaspoon Dijon mustard; 3 tablespoons tarragon vinegar; 8 tablespoons oil; 1 raw egg; 1 finely chopped garlic clove.

Mix thoroughly.

TNT Salad — Tomato and Thyme

Heap romaine lettuce in salad bowl; add garlicked squares of whole grain bread; add two sliced tomatoes; add several paper-thin slices of onion separated into rings. Add 1 tablespoon tarragon. Dress with olive oil, pepper, and vinegar.

Sauce for Fish

2 tablespoons butter; 1 green onion; ½ clove garlic; 1 tablespoon minced parsley; ¼ teaspoon thyme; ¼ teaspoon marjoram; ½ teaspoon sage.

Melt butter, mince in onion and garlic. Cook gently 5 minutes. Add parsley and other herbs. Stir, cook 5 minutes more. Mix well. Pour over fish before serving.

Sprouts

When your nutritional training wheels are off and you have made wholesome diet changes, when you appreciate the value of supplements, when you are involved in a mild exercise program, and when you want to reach a higher feel-good level of wellness, sprouting is the next step. Again, variety is recommended. Sprouting a half dozen or more different seeds and beans takes less than thirty minutes a day, but supplies you with a marvelous fresh salad always at the ready, comprised of foods literally growing until the very minute you are consuming them.

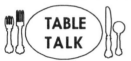

White blood cells increase after eating cooked food. These cells are on the defensive! *This does not occur after a raw food meal.* So much for the cozy smell of foods in the oven. As though to compensate, however, raw food abounds with other sensory messages.

Red beet crystals

The rich, sweet, pungent red root of the beet is a wizard's brew of important nutrients. I am especially fond of this supplement because it can disguise the not-so-pleasant tasting liquid supplement blends (like a potassium potion, for example).

One of the problems with beets is that they require a lot of cooking. Vitamin B_6, so critical to most of the beneficial actions of the nutrients in beets (and for potassium metabolism), is sensitive to high temperatures. Since beets are usually boiled for anywhere from thirty minutes to two hours (at 212 degrees F), it's safe to say that a large portion of the original B_6 is gone. Canned beets are subjected to even higher temperatures. Crystallized beets, dissolved in water, capture the sweetness of beets, retain the nutrients, and make any other nutrient mixture palatable.

FOOD DEHYDRATION

Look at any food chart listing potassium content, and you will notice that dried foods are in the lead. Here's a brief summary:

Potassium content,
milligrams per 100 grams edible portion:

Soybean, dried	1677
Lima bean, dried	1529
Banana, dried	1477
Hot red pepper, dried	1201
Mung bean, dried	1028
Pea, dried	1005
Pinto bean, dried	984
Apricot, dried	979
Peach, dried	950
Prune, dehydrated	940
Chickpea, dried	779
Lentil, dried	790
Prune, dried	694
Fig, dried	640
Coconut meat, dried	588
Apple, dried	569

Now consider:
- comparisons of the potassium content of dried foods with those listed in the food charts, pages 155-164
- reference already made to commercial dried fruits and vegetables coated with sulphites
- the fact that chips of all kinds are loaded with salt.

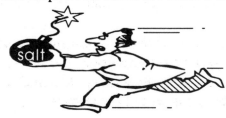

There is a solution! Believe it or not, you can compete with the various and sundry chips in today's marketplace. The answer is *home dehydration*. Dried *fruit is* common in our culture. Extend the same principle to other foods, and you're in for taste (and nutrition) treats.

What to dry? Sweet potatoes, zucchini (the first two are my favorites), tomatoes, onions, beets, green or red peppers, mushrooms, mung, wheat and lentil sprouts. And leftover foods of all kinds. You can make fruit roll-ups, cookies, "candy," crackers, chips, granola, yogurt, jerky — all without fat, salt, sugars, additives, preservatives or calories of commerical "natural" snacks. Books abound with ideas. For example, placing a cup of dried apple slices in the blender with a cup of water makes instant applesauce. And cantaloupe and watermelon slices become candy-like when dried.

How to dry? You can purchase a wonderful drying chamber that retails for around $100 (a lifetime investment), or you can make one using your oven with an extension cord and light bulb, but then your oven is tied up for 24 to 36 hours. An investment in a dehydrator (which, by the way, is an attractive accoutrement in your kitchen) pays for itself very quickly. Consider how little you get for your money when you purchase snack foods.

Although drying does not replace fresh food, it is also a way to preserve food and is most definitely a replacement for the common chips, pretzels, and other fried, roasted, sweetened and *salted* snacks. Drying does retain more nutritional value than toasting, roasting, steaming, baking or frying because the temperatures are so low (approximately 95° to 125°F).

If you have young children, I consider a drying chamber a necessity. If you want to improve your own sodium-potassium pumping efficiency without being deprived of "goody" snacks, home dehydrating is part of the answer.

WHAT OTHER THINGS *SHOULDN'T* YOU DO?

DON'T "DO" SUGAR

Enough has been written about one of the most highly processed substances in the food industry for you to know that sugar invites ill winds. Suffice it to say that it takes an entire sugar beet to yield only one teaspoon of sugar as you know it. Obviously, many nutrients go down the drain with the fiber and other constituents not utilized. No doubt, you already know the consequences. But what about sugar as it pertains to potassium?

➤*Journal of Human Nutrition and Dietetics*, 1991: If a diet is borderline in adequacy, then a high sugar diet reduces the intakes of other nutrients to below recommended daily levels.[88]

➤*Journal of Bone and Mineral*, 1990: Urinary mineral loss has been shown to occur after sugar ingestion.[89]

➤*Membrane Biochemistry*, 1989: Studies reveal that glucose suppresses the mobilization of potassium, interfering with the outward transport of this element.[90]

DON'T "DO" FATTY FOODS

When they were given a high-fat diet, a significant decrease of sodium-potassium activity occurred in cell membranes of an experimental group of test animals with respect to the controls.[91]

DON'T "DO" CAFFEINE (WELL, TRY NOT TO)

Coffee consumption is positively correlated with blood pressure among women.[92,93] One to two hours after caffeine ingestion, heart rate *and* blood pressure go up. An increase in urinary potassium is observed within one hour.[94,95] Increased urinary potassium excretion, caused by caffeine, is not in your best health interest.[96]

DON'T "DO" BURNED FATS AND RANCID OILS

Oxidized, burned, rancid, and/or artificially altered fats and oils are dietary factors that can cause a lot of damage. The real significance of dietary cholesterol is still surrounded by controversy, and it may be many years before these issues are settled. Meanwhile, I consider burned fats and rancid oils, both saturated and unsaturated, to be far more dangerous than cholesterol. Such substances can wreck havoc with cell membrane function, which, in turn, affects sodium-potassium metabolism.

You can avoid nutrition, but nutrition won't avoid you.

SUMMARY

Your own self-healing force commands breathless admiration. All you need to do is supply the armamentarium.

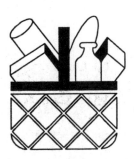

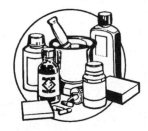

EPILOGUE

*in which Diana makes lifestyle changes
and is no longer
tired, so tired, dead tired.*

DIANA PULLS TOGETHER

(The following is a case history from the files of Richard A. Kunin, M.D., who practices medical nutrition and health medicine in San Francisco.)

The doctors found nothing wrong with Diana, and suggested she learn to relax. When she related her history of minor ailments and severe headaches, she was told to "live with it."But Diana was lucky. A friend recommended a nutrition-oriented physician.

Diana had headaches since she was four years of age. By age eight, she would come home every day after school with headache, nausea, red eyes, and blurry vision. After an hour's nap, she was better and as she advanced in years the headaches became less frequent but still might last a minimum of three hours, and sometimes all day.

Diana's bad attacks were accompanied by nausea, vomiting and other characteristics of migraine. The pain was usually located above her left eye and temple to the back of her head, and was often accompanied by scotoma — blurring of the right half of her visual field.

In addition to migraine, she complained of milder tension head-aches and spells of weakness that were relieved by eating. Severe menstrual cramps kept her at home for two days a month. Despite the magnitude of pain, dysmenorrhea and migraine, she did not take analgesic medications, not even an aspirin because of her strong belief in the Christian Science faith. Her mother had similar, though less frequent, headaches, so one would suspect a hereditary factor.

Physical examination was normal. Her lymph nodes were not enlarged, tongue was not coated, and her teeth were free of mercury amalgams. Blood pressure was normal, so she was not likely suffering from intestinal malabsorption — despite her complaining of bloat after meals. It is also unlikely that she had low sodium or low adrenal activity, either of which drop blood pressure. On the other hand, the glucose tolerance test showed a flat curve, which might have been due to excessive insulin response.

Unfortunately, insulin levels were not measured. The sugar solution given with her glucose tolerance test relieved her tension headache for an hour; then headache pain began to come and go and she was unable to concentrate on the book she was reading after four hours into the five-hour test.

Laboratory tests were normal; however, computer analysis of her diet showed deficiency in potassium, magnesium and calcium. The computer also showed only a moderate sodium intake or her symptoms might have been even worse because her low intake of vegetables was a tip-off to low potassium intake.

Her symptoms of headache, spells of weakness, and low mood were also suggestive of low blood sugar, a condition that further depletes potassium. Diana kept her food intake at only 1300 calories in an endless struggle to lose weight. She aspired to be ten pounds less than the 130 pounds that graced her 5'7" frame. She ate breakfast only half the time, and then it was only a small glass of juice and a slice of toast. Soft drinks, however, ran her sugar up to an average of 11 teaspoonsful daily and 180 "empty" calories.

Supplemental potassium gave her immediate and almost total relief of headache, a relief made more complete by the addition of magnesium — which reduced the intensity of her dysmenorrhea as well. At follow-up two years later, she reported that her headaches now came only after menses, and they cleared up after taking extra vitamins B_2 and B_6. If a headache did begin to build, an extra dose of potassium supplement (500 mg) would prevent progression and end it within an hour. Menstrual cramps were still an occasional problem, but much less than before treatment.

Why did potassium work so well? In the first place, it was deficient in her diet and made worse by low blood sugar, which commonly aggravates headache. Potassium is depleted by low blood sugar because of over-activity of insulin. This sugar-regulating hormone drives sugar into cells but uses up potassium in the process. Thus a latent potassium deficiency can become symptomatic under the influence of insulin-stimulating foods, such as sweets.

In short, the impact of hypoglycemia is to deplete potassium and thus permit increased cellular sodium and calcium, which can cause muscle spasm in muscles of the blood vessels that contract during migraine. Potassium supplementation is an important part of the dietary treatment of low blood sugar, with or without headache.

You might be interested to know that low potassium also interferes with removal of ammonia from cells, thus permitting toxic build-up to occur. One of the most sensitive indicators of ammonia excess is headache. In those who get a headache on a high protein diet, such as the weight control diet that Diana followed, low potassium is likely to be the problem behind the seeming intolerance of protein.

Richard A. Kunin, M.D.
San Francisco, CA

•

After reading this book, it is my hope that you come away with the knowledge that your metabolism can only work successfully in a stable genetic frame. If you don't want to succumb to disease, you have to adapt your nutritional behavior to its tolerances.

High technology has allowed us to delve more deeply into the dynamics of how we function, finding richer and more exciting processes at work — processes which take place within a time scale of milliseconds, yet very seriously affect our health. The results of these findings, however, often do not get translated into *Table Talk*; into meaningful applicable how-to suggestions.

When rainbow trout are placed in sea water with a higher-than-normal salinity, the effect of vitamin B_6 deficiencies are exacerbated. B_6 deficiency in humans is becoming a more serious problem. Could our imbalanced sodium-potassium ratio play a role? And who knows what other as yet undetected biological functions go awry because of the tampering of our foodways?

Yes, the sophistication of crisis medicine in the United States knows no equal. But when it comes to nutrient regulation, immune system enhancement, and especially degenerative disease, our country's establishment treatment leaves much to be desired. Our medical community has not yet ascertained that interfering with natural processes is at the very least a trade-off, and at worst creates more liability than debit.

"Is there another way?" That's the question I have learned to ask our medical experts. *"Is there another way to increase organ reserve? Is there another way to slow the aging process? Is there another way to prevent menopausal symptoms? To relieve headaches? To keep bones from thinning? To stimulate growth hormone, avoid high blood pressure, or eliminate fatigue?"*

The "other way" is not always easy, but neither is it impossible. Because of the difficulties in instituting lifestyle change, I suggest the use of quality supplements along with learning how to improve your eating habits and, of course, a regular exercise agenda. A sensible program integrates the information currently available into a rational whole — into "Table Talk."

Diana had test after test, until an astute physician recognized extremely sluggish sodium-potassium pump activity. This affected many aspects of Diana's life, including her ability to handle stress. A few sessions with a nutrition counselor, an exercise regimen, and the addition of safe supplements turned Diana's life around

SO FAR, THE ONLY THING THAT HAS CONTRIBUTED TO HEALTHY LONGEVITY IS NUTRITION.

HOW TO USE THE FOOD TABLES

The pages that follow list the sodium and potassium contents of many common foods. The first two columns — *Sodium and Potassium per 100 grams* — list the concentration of these elements in the foods. (100 grams is about four ounces, or about "a fistful.")

The next two columns are the all-important ratios. (Note that the standard chemical abbreviations are used here: Na for sodium and K for potassium.) Foods with a high sodium/potassium ratio, as we now know, are damaging to your health if eaten in quantity. High numbers in the Na/K column are bad. But the potassium/sodium ratio, which is simply the inverse of the sodium/potassium ratio, shows the good side of the relationship between these two elements. A higher number in the K/Na column means that the food is that much more valuable in offsetting the effects of too much sodium. Foods with very high potassium/sodium ratios are good for you!

Note the trend — practically all foods in their natural form have a reasonably high potassium/sodium ratio, and quite a few are extremely high. Almost all highly processed foods, on the other hand, are just the opposite.

The last three columns are for milligram-counters. By looking up the amount of sodium and potassium per serving, and the serving size on which these numbers are based, you can keep track of your actual consumption of sodium and potassium, and make some rational decisions about your own eating patterns.

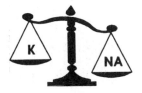

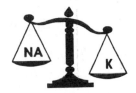

GRAINS AND GRAIN PRODUCTS

PRODUCTS	mg per 100 grams		Na/K	K/Na	mg per serving		serving
	potassium	sodium	(bad)	(good)	potassium	sodium	size
bran flakes	428	628	1	1	485	712	4 oz.
brown rice, cooked	70	282	4	0	79	320	4 oz.
corn flakes	92	968	11	0	104	1098	4 oz.
farina, instant	13	188	14	0	30	426	8 oz.
French bread	90	580	6	0	26	164	1 oz.
graham crackers	386	671	2	1	109	190	1 oz.
hamburger/hot dog buns	93	507	5	0	53	287	2 oz.
macaroni & cheese	120	543	5	0	272	1232	8 oz.
oat meal, cooked	61	218	4	0	138	495	8 oz.
pancakes	244	464	2	1	554	1053	8 oz.
pizza	131	703	5	0	296	1594	8 oz.
pretzels	130	1683	13	0	147	1909	4 oz.
shredded wheat	346	3	0	115	393	3	4 oz.
spaghetti with meat sauce	268	407	2	1	608	924	8 oz.
toasted wheat germ	948	2	0	474	1075	2	4 oz.
waffles	145	477	3	0	330	1083	8 oz.
wheat bran	1276	9	0	142	1447	10	4 oz.
white bread	100	540	5	0	28	153	1 oz.
white rice, cooked	28	374	13	0	32	424	4 oz.
whole wheat flour	370	3	0	123	105	1	1 oz.

FRUITS	mg per 100 grams		Na/K	K/Na	mg per serving		serving
	potassium	sodium	(bad)	(good)	potassium	sodium	size
apples	110	1	0	143	249	2	8 oz.
apricots, dried	979	26	0	38	1110	29	4 oz.
apricots, uncooked	282	34	0	8	319	38	4 oz.
avocado	604	4	0	151	1370	9	8 oz.
banana	370	1	0	370	839	2	8 oz.
blueberries	81	1	0	113	92	1	4 oz.
cantaloupe	251	12	0	21	569	27	8 oz.
cherries	191	2	0	96	217	2	4 oz.
dates, dried	650	1	0	650	737	1	4 oz.
figs, dried	638	34	0	19	724	39	4 oz.
grapefruit	148	1	0	133	336	3	8 oz.
grapes, green, seedless	110	4	0	28	249	9	8 oz.
olives, canned	27	757	28	0	30	859	4 oz.
orange	200	1	0	200	454	2	8 oz.
peach	205	1	0	205	233	1	4 oz.
pears, canned	90	1	0	90	102	1	4 oz.
pears, uncooked	130	2	0	65	147	2	4 oz.
pineapple	146	1	0	146	330	2	8 oz.
strawberries	164	1	0	164	186	1	4 oz.
watermelon	100	1	0	100	227	2	8 oz.

MEATS

	mg per 100 grams		Na/K	K/Na	mg per serving		serving
	potassium	sodium	(bad)	(good)	potassium	sodium	size
bacon, broiled or fried	236	1021	4	0	268	1158	4 oz.
bacon, Canadian	432	2555	6	0	490	2897	4 oz.
bacon, uncooked	250	1400	6	0	284	1588	4 oz.
beef liver, cooked	380	184	0	2	862	418	8 oz.
beef, pot roast or chuck roast	370	60	0	6	839	136	8 oz.
beef, uncooked	280	55	0	5	318	62	4 oz.
bologna	230	1302	6	0	522	2952	8 oz.
chicken chow mein	189	287	2	1	429	651	8 oz.
chicken liver, cooked	151	61	0	2	342	138	8 oz.
chicken, broiled	274	66	0	4	621	150	8 oz.
corned beef	150	1740	12	0	340	3946	8 oz.
frankfurter	217	1084	5	0	492	2459	8 oz.
hamburger	451	47	0	10	1022	107	8 oz.
ham, cured, roast	332	718	2	0	753	1628	8 oz.
lamb, roast leg	290	70	0	4	657	159	8 oz.
pork chops, roast	568	60	0	9	1288	136	8 oz.
pork, uncooked	270	65	0	4	306	74	4 oz.
steak, T-bone, porterhouse, rib	4	53	13	0	9	120	8 oz.
turkey, roast dark meat	398	99	0	4	902	224	8 oz.
turkey, roast light meat	411	82	0	5	932	186	8 oz.

MEATS (continued)

	mg per 100 grams		Na/K	K/Na	mg per serving		serving
	potassium	sodium	(bad)	(good)	potassium	sodium	size
TV dinner, meat loaf	115	393	3	0	261	891	8 oz.
TV dinner, turkey	250	568	2	0	568	1288	8 oz.
veal cutlet, broiled	527	54	0	10	1195	123	8 oz.

FISH AND SEAFOOD

	mg per 100 grams		Na/K	K/Na	mg per serving		serving
	potassium	sodium	(bad)	(good)	potassium	sodium	size
crabmeat, canned	110	850	8	0	249	1928	8 oz.
flounder, baked	596	241	0	2	1352	546	8 oz.
haddock, smoked	190	790	4	0	431	1792	8 oz.
haddock, uncooked	300	120	0	3	680	272	8 oz.
halibut, broiled	533	136	0	4	1209	308	8 oz.
kelp	5273	3007	1	2	1495	852	1 oz.
salmon, sockeye, canned	342	520	2	1	777	1179	8 oz.
sardines, canned in oil	558	508	1	1	1265	1152	8 oz.
shrimp, cooked	228	185	1	1	517	420	8 oz.
tuna, canned in oil, drained	296	790	3	0	671	1792	8 oz.

qq

SAUCES AND CONDIMENTS

	mg per 100 grams		Na/K	K/Na	mg per serving		serving
	potassium	sodium	(bad)	(good)	potassium	sodium	size
blackstrap molasses	2925	95	0	31	829	27	1 oz.
French salad dressing	80	1373	17	0	23	389	1 oz.
iodized table salt	4	38760	9690	0	1	10988	1 oz.
Italian salad dressing	15	2093	140	0	4	593	1 oz.
light molasses	915	15	0	61	259	4	1 oz.
maple syrup	175	15	0	12	50	4	1 oz.
mustard	133	1250	9	0	38	354	1 oz.
soy sauce	367	7327	20	0	104	2077	1 oz.
tomato catsup	365	688	2	1	103	195	1 oz.

JUICES

	mg per 100 grams		Na/K	K/Na	mg per serving		serving
	potassium	sodium	(bad)	(good)	potassium	sodium	size
apple juice	101	1	0	101	230	2	8 oz.
grapefruit juice	153	3	0	61	347	6	8 oz.
lemon juice	564	1	0	564	160	0	1 oz.
orange juice, fresh	200	1	0	200	454	2	8 oz.
orange juice, frozen concentrate	286	2	0	181	649	4	8 oz.
tomato juice	227	200	1	1	515	454	8 oz.

EGGS AND DAIRY PRODUCTS

	mg per 100 grams		Na/K	K/Na	mg per serving		serving
	potassium	sodium	(bad)	(good)	potassium	sodium	size
cheese, American or cheddar	82	700	9	0	93	794	4 oz.
cheese, creamed cottage	85	229	3	0	193	519	8 oz.
cheese, parmesan	150	732	5	0	170	830	4 oz.
egg, raw, boiled, or poached	130	122	1	1	74	69	2 oz.
milk, human	50	17	0	3	113	38	8 oz.
milk, skim	142	50	0	3	322	113	8 oz.
skim milk	145	76	1	2	329	173	8 oz.
yogurt, low-fat	143	51	0	3	325	116	8 oz.

NUTS, SEEDS, NUT BUTTER

	mg per 100 grams		Na/K	K/Na	mg per serving		serving
	potassium	sodium	(bad)	(good)	potassium	sodium	size
almonds, roasted and salted	773	198	0	4	876	224	4 oz.
cashews, unsalted	464	15	0	31	526	17	4 oz.
cashews, salted	464	200	0	2	526	227	4 oz.
peanut butter	627	607	1	1	711	688	4 oz.
peanuts, roasted, salted	673	418	1	2	764	474	4 oz.
sunflower seeds	920	30	0	31	1043	34	4 oz.
walnuts	460	3	0	153	522	3	4 oz.

VEGETABLES

	mg per 100 grams		Na/K	K/Na	mg per serving		serving
	potassium	sodium	(bad)	(good)	potassium	sodium	size
artichoke, cooked	301	30	0	10	341	34	4 oz.
artichoke, uncooked	430	43	0	10	488	49	4 oz.
asparagus, cooked	183	1	0	183	52	0	1 oz.
asparagus, uncooked	278	2	0	148	79	1	1 oz.
baked potatoes, with skin	503	4	0	126	1141	9	8 oz.
beets, boiled	208	43	0	5	236	49	4 oz.
broccoli, cooked	267	10	0	27	303	11	4 oz.
Brussels sprouts, cooked	273	1	0	273	310	1	4 oz.
cabbage, boiled	130	230	2	1	147	261	4 oz.
cabbage, uncooked	390	7	0	56	442	8	4 oz.
carrots, raw	341	47	0	7	387	53	4 oz.
cauliflower, raw	295	13	0	23	335	15	4 oz.
celery, raw	342	126	0	3	388	143	4 oz.
corn, canned or cooked	97	236	2	0	110	268	4 oz.
cauliflower, steamed	206	9	0	23	233	10	4 oz.
creamed corn, cooked	97	236	2	0	110	268	4 oz.
cucumber, raw, unpeeled	160	6	0	27	181	7	4 oz.
eggplant, steamed	214	2	0	107	243	2	4 oz.
French fried potatoes	862	6	0	144	1954	14	8 oz.
garbanzos, raw	797	26	0	31	904	29	4 oz.

VEGETABLES

(continued)	mg per 100 grams		Na/K (bad)	K/Na (good)	mg per serving		serving size
	potassium	sodium			potassium	sodium	
garlic	530	19	0	28	150	5	1 oz.
green beens, cooked	151	4	0	38	171	5	4 oz.
green lima beens, raw	650	2	0	325	737	2	4 oz.
green peas, canned	96	236	2	0	109	268	4 oz.
green peas, fresh cooked	196	1	0	196	222	1	4 oz.
green peas, frozen	135	115	1	1	153	130	4 oz.
green peas, uncooked	340	1	0	340	386	1	4 oz.
lettuce, iceberg	175	9	0	19	198	10	4 oz.
mung bean sprouts, raw	224	5	0	45	254	6	4 oz.
mushrooms, cooked or canned	197	400	2	0	223	454	4 oz.
onions, cooked	110	7	0	16	125	8	4 oz.
parsley, raw	407	25	0	16	115	7	1 oz.
pickles, dill or sour	200	1428	7	0	227	1619	4 oz.
potato salad	296	480	2	1	335	544	4 oz.
red kidney beans, canned	264	3	0	88	299	3	4 oz.
romaine or leaf lettuce	264	9	0	29	299	10	4 oz.
sauerkraut, canned	140	747	5	0	159	847	4 oz.
spinach, steamed	324	50	0	6	367	57	4 oz.
vegetables, mixed frozen	191	53	0	4	217	60	4 oz.

VEGETABLES

(continued)	mg per 100 grams		Na/K	K/Na	mg per serving		serving
	potassium	sodium	(bad)	(good)	potassium	sodium	size
squash, cooked	141	1	0	141	320	2	8 oz.
squash, uncooked	202	1	0	202	458	2	8 oz.
succotash, frozen	38	246	6	0	43	279	4 oz.
sweet potato, baked	300	12	0	25	340	14	4 oz.
sweet potato, candied	190	42	0	5	216	48	4 oz.
swiss chard, steamed	321	86	0	4	364	98	4 oz.
tomato paste, canned	888	38	0	23	1007	43	4 oz.
tomato puree, canned	426	399	1	1	966	905	8 oz.
tomato, canned	217	130	1	2	492	295	8 oz.
tomato, uncooked	244	1	0	244	277	1	4 oz.

SOUPS

	mg per 100 grams		Na/K	K/Na	mg per serving		serving
	potassium	sodium	(bad)	(good)	potassium	sodium	size
chicken noodle soup	23	408	18	0	53	925	8 oz.
ministrone	123	406	3	0	279	921	8 oz.
split pea soup	110	384	3	0	249	871	8 oz.

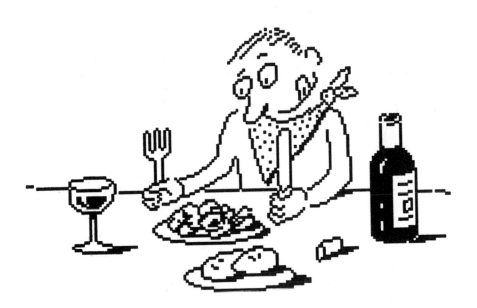

LET'S EAT!

REFERENCES

PROLOGUE

[1] Fairweather DS; Campbell AJ. "Diagnostic accuracy. The effects of multiple aetiology and the degradation of information in old age."*Jnl of Royal Col of Phys of London*, 1991 Apr, 25(2):105.

[2] Dardick Iet al."A rev of the proliferative capacity of major salivary glands and the relationship to current concepts of neoplasia in salivary glands." *Oral Surg, Oral Med, Oral Path*, 1990 Jan, 69(1):53-67.

[3] Ji LL et al."Antiox enzyme response to selenium deficiency in rat myocardium" *Jnl of the Amer Col of Nutr*, 1992 Feb, 11(1):79-86.

[4] Wolff MR et al."Alterations in left ventricular mechanics, energetics, and contractile reserve in exper heart failure."*Circ Res*, 1992 Mar, 70(3):516-29.

[5] Toloza EM; Lam M; Diamond J."Nutrient extraction by cold-exposed mice: a test of digestive safety margins."*Amer Jnl of Phys*, 1991 Oct, 261(4 Pt 1):G608-20.

[6] Riecken EO; Balzer T.["Physiologic and pathologic age related changes in the small intestine."]*Fortschritte der Medizin*, 1990 Nov 30, 108(34):654-6.

[7] Pinsky MR; Schlichtig R."Regional oxygen delivery in oxygen Supy-dependent states."*Intensive Care Med*, 1990, 16 Sup 2:S169-71.

[8] Wallach S."Availability of body magnesium during magnesium deficiency."*Magnesium*, 1988, 7(5-6):262.

[9] Lee HC et al."Compensatory adaption to partial pancreatectomy in the rat."*Endoc*, 1989 Mar, 124(3):1571.

[10] Rogov VA.["The renal functional reserve in the nephrotic syndrome."]*Terapevticheskii Arkhiv*, 1990, 62(6):55-8.

[11] Fries JF; Crapo LM. *Vitality and Aging* (SF: WH Freeman & Co., 1981), p 32.

[12] Sophocles, Oedipus at Colonus (406 BC)

[13] Roe DA."Ger Nutr."*Clin in Ger Med*, 1990 May, 6):319-34.

[14] D Rudman, "Growth Hormone, Body Composition, and Aging," *Jnl of the Amer Ger Soc* 33 (1985):800-7.

[15] Morimoto S; Ogihara T.["Physl and pathological aging and electrolyte metabolism."]*Nippon Ronen Igakkai Zasshi. Jap Jnl of Gers*, 1991 May, 28:325-30.

[16] Mimran A.[Renal function and aging].*Neph*, 1990,11:275

[17] Gillen-Hansen P.*It's Never Too Late! Restore the Youthful Look of Your Skin Without Drugs or Surgery*, 1990, p 19.

PART I

[1] Smith H W. *Fish to Philosopher: Story of Our Int Environment*, CIBA Pharm Products, Inc., Summit, NY.

[2] Rettig R; Ganten D; Luft FC. *Salt and Hypert*, 1988, Springer Verlag, Berlin.

[3] Maxwell MH et al.*Clin Disorders of Fluid and Electrolyte Metabolism*, 1987, McGraw-Hill Book Co, NY.

[4] "Cardiac Failure," Bine R, in *Hum Nutr: A Comprehensive Treatise*, eds Alfin-Slater, RB; Kritchevsky, D. (NY: Plenum Press, 1979), p 174-5.

[5] Contreras RJ. "Sodium deprivation alters neural responses to gustatory stimuli."*Jnl of Gen Phys*, 1979, 73:569.

[6] O'Dell BL."Min interactions relevant to nutrient requirements."*Jnl of Nutr*, 1989 Dec, 119(12 Sup):1832-8.

[7] Linas SL."Potassium: weighing the evidence for Supation."*Hospi Prac*, 1988 Dec 15, 23(12):73, 83-4, 86.

[8] Krakoff, I. "Is reduction of dietary salt a treatment for hypert?" *Amer Jnl of Public Health*, 1991, 41

[9] McCarron DA. "The integrated effects of electrolytes on blood pressure."*The Nutr Report*, 1991 Aug, 9(8):57,62,64.

[10] Roe DA. *Drug Induced Nutral Deficiencies* (Westpt, Conn: The Avi Publ Co, Inc, 1978), p 132.

[11] Werbach MR. *Nutral Influences on Illness* (New Canaan, Conn: Keats Publ, Inc, 1988), p 492.

[12] Sangiori GB et al. "Serum potassium levels, red-blood-cell potassium and alterations of the repolarization phase of electrocardiography in old subjects." *Age Aging*, 1984, 13:309.

[13] Ibid.

[14] *Circ*, 1988, 78:951.

[15] *AJCN*, 191979, 32:2410.

[16] *Brit Med Jnl*, 1986, 292:1697

[17] Sangiori GB et al. Op cit.

[18] *Nutr Res Revs* 1990, 3:101.

[19] Walker WF. "Nutr after injury. In *World Rev of Nutr and Dietetics*, 1974, 19:173-204.

[20] *AJCN*, 1988 47:50.

[21] Sangiori GB et al. Op cit.

[22] Smith, TJ; Edelman, IS. "The role of sodium transport in thyroid thermogenesis." *Fed Proc*, 1979, 38:2150.

[23] Luft FC. "Sodium, Chloride, and Potassium," in *Present Knowledge in Nutr*, 6th ed [[[etc.

[24] Ikeda U; et al."Aldosterone-mediated regulation of Na+, K(+)-ATPase gene expression in adult and neonatal rat cardiocytes"*Jnl of Biol Chem*, 1991 Jun 25, 266(18):12058-66.

PART II

[1] Weinberger MH. "Can essential hypert be subclassified with respect to mechanism?" *Hypert*, 1991 Sep, 18(3 Sup):I82-6.

[2] Horan MJ."Implications for res and policy in the treatment of hypert:Med considerations." *Hypert*, 1989 May, 13(5 Sup):I164-6.

[3] Stamler J. "Blood pressure and high blood pressure. Aspects of risk." *Hypert*, 1991 Sep, 18(3 Sup):I95-107.

[4] Tobian L."Protecting arteries against hypertensive injury." *Clin and Exper Hypert*. Part A, Theory and Practice, 1992,14(1-2):35-43.

[5] Krishna GG."Potassium depletion exacerbates essential Hypert."*Ann of Int Med*, 1991 Jul 15, 115:77-83.

[6] Speckmann; Brink. *Jnl of the Amer Dietetic Assoc*, 1967, 51:517.

[7] Kamen B; Kamen S. *The Kamen Plan for Total Nutr During Pregnancy* (Norwalk, Conn: Appleton-Century-Crofts, 1981), p 147.

[8] Aloia et al. "Relationship of menopause to skeletal and muscle mass." *AJCN*, 1991, 53:1378-83.

[9] Lemann J Jr; Gray RW."Idiopathic hypercalciuria." *Jnl of Urology*, 1989 Mar, 141(3 Pt 2):715.

[10] Scala J. *High Blood Pressure Relief Diet* (NY: Penguin, 1990), p 49.

[11] Stamler J."Blood pressure and high blood pressure. Aspects of risk." *Hypert*, 1991 Sep, 18(3 Sup):I95-107.

[12] Oboler SK et al. "Leg symptoms in outpatient veterans."*W Jnl of Med*, 1991 Sep, 155:256-9.

[13] Hegsted DM. "A perspective on reducing salt intake."*Hypert,* 1991 Jan, 17(1 Sup):I201-4.

[14] Kotchen TA; Kotchen JM; Boegehold MA."Nutr and Hypert Prev." *Hypert*, 1991 Sep, 18(3 Sup):I115-20.

[15] Suki WN. "Dietary potassium and blood pressure." *Kidney Inter*, 1988, 34 (Sup 25):S175-6.

[16] Leckie BJ."High blood pressure: hunting the genes." *Bioessays*, 1992 Jan, 14(1):37-41.

[17] *Brit Med Jnl*, 1991, 302:815.

[18] Elmer PJ et al. "Dietary sodium reduction for Hypert Prev and treatment." *Hypert*, 1991 Jan, 17(1 Sup):I182.

[19] Mattiasson I; Berntorp K; Lindgarde F. "Insulin resistance and Na+/K(+)-ATPase in hypertensive women: a difference in mechanism depending on the level of glucose tolerance." *Clin Sci*, 1992 Jan, 82(1):105-11.

[20] Gettes LS."Electrolyte abnormalities underlying lethal and ventricular arrhythmias." *Circ*, 1992 Jan, 85(1 Sup):I70-6.

[21] Fitzovich DE; et al. "Chronic hypokalemia and the left ventricular responses to epinephrine and preload. *Jnl of the Amer Col of Card*, 1991 Oct, 18(4):1105-11.

[22] Pogorelov A et al." Study of potassium deficiency in cardiac muscle: quantitative X-ray microanalysis and cryotechniques." *Jnl of Microscopy*, 1991 May, 162 (Pt 2):255-69.

[23] Joossens JV."Trends in systolic blood pressure, 24-hour sodium excretion, and stroke mortality in the elderly in Belgium." *Amer Jnl of Med*, 1991 Mar, 90(3A):5S-11S.

[24] Horie R; et al."Blood pressure levels in the elderly with or without Nutral intervention." *Jnl of Cardiov Pharm*, 1990, 16 Sup 8:S57-8.

[25] SE Kjeldsen, "Increased erythrocyte magnesium in never treated essential hypert," *Amer Jnl of Hypert*, 1990, 3:573.

[26] Bruce NG et al."Casual urine concentrations of sodium, potassium, and creatine in population studies of blood pressure. *Jnl of Hum Hypert*, 1990 Dec, 4(6):597-602.

[27] Krishna GG; Miller E; Kapoor S. "Increased blood pressure during potassium depletion in normotensive men." *NEJM*, 1989, 320:1177-82.

[28] *AJCN*, 1981, 34:527.

[29] Halpern SL. *Quick Reference to Clin Nutr: A Guide for Phys* (Phil: JB Lippencott Co., 1979), p 67.

[30] Mtabaji JP; et al."Diet and Hypert in Tanzania." *Jnl of Cardiov Pharm*, 1990, 16 Sup 8:S3-5.

[31] Del Pozo G; Davalos P; Yamori Y. "Cardiov risk factors in two Ecuadorian urban and rural populations. The Ecuadorian-Japan Cooperative CARDIAC Study Group. " *Jnl of Cardiov Pharm*, 1990, 16 Sup 8:S24-5.

[32] Abdulla M; Behbehani A; Dashti H. "Dietary intake and bioavailability of trace elements."*Biol Trace Element Res*, 1989 Jul-Sep, 21:173-8.

[33] Cocchioni M et al. ["Daily intake of macro and trace elements in the diet. 4. Sodium, potassium, calcium, and magnesium."] *Annali di Igiene*, 1989 Sep-Oct, 1(5):923-42.

[34] Liu LS; et al. "Variability of urinary sodium and potassium excretion in north Chinese men."*Jnl of Hypert*, 1987, 5:331-5.

[35] Lijnen P; et al."Erythrocyte concentrations and transMemb fluxes of sodium and potassium in essential Hypert: role of intrinsic and Envir factors." *Cardiov Drugs and Ther*, 1990 Mar, 4 Sup 2:321-33.

[36] Editorial. "Hypert—in black and white." *Lancet*, 1992, 339:28-29.

[37] Pfeiffer CC; Mailloux RJ."Hypert: heavy metals, useful cations and melanin as a possible repository," *Med Hypothesis*, 1988 Jun, 26(2):125-30.

[38] Dustan HP. "Growth factors and racial differences in severity of Hypert and renal diseases." *Lancet*, May 1992, 339:1339-42.

[39] Pfeiffer CC; Mailloux RJ. Op cit.

[40] Anastos K et al."Hypert in women: what is really known? Women's Caucus, Working Group on Women's Health of the Soc of Gen Int Med." *Ann of Int Med*, 1991 Aug 15, 115:287-93.

[41] Weinberger MH. Op cit.

[42] Branche GC et al."Improving compliance in an inner-city hypertensive patient population." *Amer Jnl of Med*, 1991 Jul 18, 91(1A):37S-41S.

[43] Gorlin R."Hypert and vascular disease in the 1990s."*Clin Card*, 1991 Aug, 14(8 Sup 4):IV1-5.

[44] Fries ED. "Should mild Hypert be treated?" *NEJM*, 1982, 307:306-9.

[45] Parish RC; Miller LJ."Adverse effects of angiotensin converting enzyme (ACE) inhibitors. An update." *Drug Safety*, 1992 Jan-Feb, 7(1):14-31.

[46] Black HR."Choosing initial Ther for Hypert. A personal view." *Hypert*, 1989 May, 13(5 Sup):I149-53.

[47] Parish RC; Miller LJ."Adverse effects of angiotensin converting enzyme (ACE)

[48] Bellin LJ. " Jones NL; Heigenhauser GJ."Factors contributing to increased muscle fatigue with beta-blockers."*Can Jnl of Phys and Pharm*, 1991 Feb, 69(2):254-61.

[49] RL; Daelemans RA; Verbraeken H."Diuretics in the treatment of Hypert." *Acta Clinica Belgica*, 1991, 46(3):165-77.

[50] *Nutr Res Revs*, 1990, 3:101.[51] Lindholm LH."Cardiov risk factors and their interactions in hypertensives." *Jnl of Hypert*. Sup, 1991 Dec, 9(3):S3-6.

[51] Lindholm LH."Cardiov risk factors and their interactions in hypertensives. " *Jnl of Hypert*. Sup, 1991 Dec, 9(3):S3-6.

[52] McKelvie RS; Jones NL; Heigenhauser GJ."Factors contributing to increased muscle fatigue with beta-blockers."*Can Jnl of Phys and Pharm*, 1991 Feb, 69(2):254-61.

[53] McKelvie RS; Jones NL; Heigenhauser GJ."Factors contributing to increased muscle fatigue with beta-blockers." *Can Jnl of Phys and Pharm*, 1991 Feb, 69(2):254-61.

[54] Wassertheil-Smoller; et al."Effect of antihypertensives on sexual function and quality of life: the TAIM Study." *Ann of Int Med*, 1991 Apr 15, 114(8):613-20.

[55] McKelvie RS; Jones NL; Heigenhauser GJ. Op cit.

[56] Schmidt GR; Schuna AA; Goodfriend TL. "Transdermal clonidine compared with hydrochlorothiazide as monoTher in elderly hypertensive males." *Jnl of Clin Pharm*, 1989 Feb, 29(2):133-9.

[57] Ibid.

[58] Kaku T et al."Dry cough in the elderly patients treated with angiotensin converting enzyme inhibitor." *Jap Jnl of Gers*, 1991 May, 28(3):365-70.

[59] O'Byrne S; Feely J. "Effects of drugs on glucose tolerance in non-insulin-dependent diabetics (Part I)" *Drugs*, 1990 Jul, 40(1):6-18.

[60] Berger BE; Warnock DG. "Clin uses and mechanisms of action of diuretic agents." In: *The Kidney* , 3rd ed., vol 1 (Brenner BM and Rector, Jr. FC, eds), pp 433-55, W B Saunders, Phil.

[61] Prisant LM et al. "Depression associated with antihypertensive drugs." *Jnl of Fam Pract*, 1991 Nov, 33(5):481-5.

[62] Dahlof C."Quality of life/subjective symptoms during beta-blocker treatment." *Scand Jnl of Primary Health Care*. Supl, 1990, 1:73.

[63] "The effects of nonpharmacologic interventions on blood pressure of persons with high normal levels. Results of the Trials of Hypert Prev, Phase I." Jama, 1992 Mar 4, 267(9):1213-20.

[64] Little P et al."A controlled trial of a low sodium, low fat, high fibre diet in treated hypert patients: effect on antihypertensive drug requirement in clin pract." *Jnl of Hum Hypert*, 1991, 5(3):175.

[65] Langford HG."Nonpharmacological Ther of Hypert. Commentary on diet and blood pressure." *Hypert*, 1989 May, 13(5 Sup):I98-102.

[66] Personal interview with Michael Rosenbaum, MD, Corte Madera, CA, May 1992.

[67] Everts ME; Retterstol K; Clausen T. "Effects of adrenaline on excitation-induced stimulation of the sodium-potassium pump in rat skeletal muscle." *Acta Phys Scan*, 1988 Oct, 134(2):189-98.

[68] Kossler F et al. ["Problems of muscular fatigue—relationship to stimulation conduction velocity and K(+) concentration"]. *Zeitschrift fur die Gesamte Hygiene und Ihre Grenzgebiete*, 1990 Jul, 36(7):354-6.

[69] Lindinger MI; Sjogaard G. "Potassium regulation during exercise and recovery." *Sports Med*, 1991 Jun, 11(6):382-401.

[70] Lindinger MI; Heigenhauser GJ. "The roles of ion fluxes in skeletal muscle fatigue." *Can Jnl of Phys and Pharm*, 1991 Feb, 69):246-53.

[71] Sjogaard G."Role of exercise-induced potassium fluxes underlying muscle fatigue: a brief Rev." *Can Jnl of Phys and Pharm*, 1991 Feb, 69(2):238-45.

[72] Kaminsky LA; Paul GL."Fluid intake during an ultramarathon running race: relationship to plasma volume and serum sodium and potassium." *Jnl of Sports Med and Phys Fitness*, 1991 Sep, 31(3):417-9.

[73] Pichard C; et al. "Intracellular potassium and Memb potential in rat muscles during malNutr and subsequent refeeding." *AJCN*, 1991 Sep, 54(3):489-98.

[74] Sjogaard G. "Role of exercise-induced potassium fluxes underlying muscle fatigue: a brief Rev." *Can Jnl of Phys and Pharm*, 1991 Feb, 69(2):238-45.

[75] Lindinger MI; Heigenhauser GJ. Op cit.

[76] Lindinger MI et al. "Blood ion regulation during repeated maximal exercise and recovery in Hums." *Amer Jnl of Phys*, 1992 Jan, 262:R126.

[77] Bystrom S; Sjogaard G."Potassium homeostasis during and following exhaustive submaximal static handgrip contractions." *Acta Phys Scan*, 1991 May, 142(1):59-66.

[78] Gullestad L; et al. "The importance of potassium and lactate for maximal exercise performance during beta blockade." *Scandinavian Jnl of Clin and Lab Invest*, 1989 Oct, 49(6):521-8.

[79] Lindinger MI; Sjogaard G. Op cit.

[80] Kjeldsen K; Norgaard A; Hau C."Exercise-induced hyperkalemia can be reduced in Hum subjects by moderate training without change in skeletal muscle Na,K-ATPase concentration." *Eur Jnl of Clin Invest*, 1990 Dec, 20(6):642-7.

[81] Sullivan PA et al. "Strenuous short-term dynamic exercise: effects on heart rate, blood pressure, potassium homeostasis, and packed cell volume in mild Hypert." *Jnl of Hypert*. Supl 1989 Dec, 7):S90.

[82] Deyhim F; Teeter RG."Sodium and potassium chloride drinking water Supation effects on acid-base balance and plasma corticosterone in broilers reared in thermoneutral and heat-distressed environments." *Poultry Sci*, 1991 Dec, 70(12):2551-3.

[83] Maughan RJ."Fluid and electrolyte loss and replacement in exercise." *Jnl of Sports Scis*, 1991 Summer, 9 Spec No:117-42.

[84] Deriaz O; et al."Hum resting energy expenditure in relation to dietary potassium." *AJCN*, 1991 Oct, 54(4):628-34.

[85] Ameen M et al."Reversal of effects of low extracellular potassium concentration on number and activity of Na+/K+ pumps in Epstein-Barr virus-transformed Hum lymphocyte cell line." *Bio Pharm*, 1992 Feb 4, 43(3):489-96.

[86] Hamlyn JM et al. "Identification and characterization of a ouabain-like compound from Hum plasma." *Proc of the National Acad of Scis of the United States of America*, 1991 Jul 15, 88:6259.

[87] Lauber M; Boni-Schnetzler M; Muller J."Potassium raises cytochrome P-45011 beta mRNA level in zona glomerulosa of rat adrenals." *Mol and Cellular Endoc*, 1990 Sep 10, 72(3):159-66.

[88] Inagami T et al. "Active and inactive renin in the adrenal." *Amer Jnl of Hypert*, 1989 Apr, 2(4):311-9.

[89] Tremblay A; et al."Regulation of rat adrenal messenger RNA and protein levels for cytochrome P-450s and adrenodoxin by dietary sodium depletion or potassium intake." *Jnl of Biol Chem*, 1991 Feb 5, 266(4):2245-51.

[90] Rosenbaum, M; Susser, M. *Solving the Puzzle of Chronic Fatigue Syndrome* (Tacoma, WA: Life Scis Press, 1992), p 78-9.

[91] Quinn SJ; Williams GH."Regulation of aldosterone secretion." *Annual Rev of Phys*, 1988, 50:409-26.

[92] Rajanna B et al."Effects of cadmium and mercury on Na(+)-K+, ATPase and uptake of 3H-dopamine in rat brain synaptosomes.
" *Archives Interes de Phys et de Biochimie*, 1990 Oct,98:291-6.

[93] Kone BC; Brenner RM; Gullans SR."Sulfhydryl-reactive heavy metals increase cell Memb K+ and Ca2+ transport in renal proximal tubule.
" *Jnl of Memb Biol*, 1990 Jan, 113(1):1-12.

[94] Rai LC et al."Effect of four heavy metals on the Biol of Nostoc muscorum." *Biol of Metals*, 1990, 2(4):229.

[95] Bertoni JM; Sprenkle PM. "Low level lead inhibits the Hum brain cation pump." *Life Scis*, 1991, 48(22):2149.

[96] Mimran A.[Renal function and aging].*Neph*, 1990, 11:275-80.

[97] Ruch S et al."Aging: stimulation rate on cardiac intracellular Na+ activity and developed tension." *Mechanisms of Ageing and Devel*, 1991 Nov 1, 60(3):303-13.

[98] Rudman D; et al. "Effects of Hum Growth Hormone in Men Over 60 Years Old." *NEJM*, 1990, 323:1-6.

[99] Vance ML. "Growth Hormone for the Elderly?" *NEJM*, July 1990, 323 (1):52-4.

[100] Flyvbjerg A; et al."Evidence that potassium deficiency induces growth retardation through reduced circulating levels of growth hormone and insulin-like growth factor I." *Metabolism: Clin and Exper*, 1991 Aug, 40(8):769-75.

[101] Gorban' EN.[Effect of Ca2+- and K+-channel blockers on ACTH-stimulated steroidogenesis of isolated adrenal glands of adult and old rats].*Fiziologicheskii Zhurnal*, 1990 Sep-Oct, 36(5):99.

[102] Adragna NC."Cation transport in vascular endothelial cells and aging." *Jnl of Memb Biol*, 1991 Dec, 124(3):285-91.

[103] Heseltine D; et al."Erythrocyte sodium, potassium and sodium fluxes with cell and subject ageing." *Clinica Chimica Acta*, 1991 Jan 31, 196(1):41-7.

[104] Akera T; Ng YC."Digitalis sensitivity of Na+,K(+)-ATPase, myocytes and the heart." *Life Scis*, 1991, 48(2):97-106.

[105] Sparrow D; et al."Methacholine airway responsiveness and 24-hour urine excretion of sodium and potassium. The Normative Aging Study." *Amer Rev of Respiratory Disease*, 1991 Sep, 144(3 Pt 1):722-5.

[106] Tosco M et al."Aging and ATPase activities in rat jejunum." *Mechanisms of Ageing and Devel*, 1990 Dec, 56(3):265-74.

[107] Adeeb N; Ton SH; Muslim N."Effect of age, weight, race and sex on blood pressure and erythrocyte sodium pump characteristics." *Clin and Exper Hypert. Part A, Theory and Practice*, 1990,12(6):1115-34.

[108] Touitou Y et al."Prevalence of magnesium and potassium deficiencies in the elderly." *Clin Chem*, 1987 Apr, 33(4):518-23.

[109] Cowar NR; Judge TG. *Jnl of the Amer Med Assoc*, October 6, 1969.

[110] Bosman GJ; Bartholomeus IG; de Grip WJ."Alzheimer's disease and cellular aging: Memb-related events as clues to primary mechanisms." *Ger*, 1991, 37(1-3):95-112.

[111] Rhodus NL; Brown J."The Assoc of xerostomia and inadequate intake in older adults." *Jnl of the Amer Dietetic Assoc*, 1990 Dec, 90(12):1688-92.

[112] Shah J; Jandhyala BS."Role of Na+,K(+)-ATPase in the centrally mediated hypotensive effects of potassium in anaesthetized rats." *Jnl of Hypert, 1991 Feb, 9(2):167-70.

[113] Webb WL; Gehi M. "Electrolyte and fluid imbalance: Neuropsychiatric manifestations." *Psychosomatics*, 1981, 22(3):199-203.

[114] Parmelee JT et al."Response of infant and adult rat choroid plexus potassium transporters to increased extracellular potassium." *Develal Brain Res*, 1991 Jun 21, 60(2):229-33.

[115] Mancini M et al."Metabolic disturbances and antihypertensive Ther." *Jnl of Hypert*. Sup, 1991 Dec, 9(3):S47.

[116] Lees GJ."Inhibition of sodium-potassium-ATPase: a potentially ubiquitous mechanism contributing to central nervous system neuroPath." *Brain Res*. Brain Res Revs, 1991 Sep-Dec, 16(3):283-300.

[117] O'Dell BL; et al."Zinc status and peripheral nerve function in guinea pigs." *Faseb Jnl*, 1990 Aug, 4(11):2919.

[118] Hokin-Neaverson M; Jefferson JW."Erythrocyte sodium pump activity in bipolar affective disorder and other psychiatric disorders." *NeuropsychoBiol*, 1989, 22(1):1-7.

[119] Mozsik GY; et al. "A Bio and pharmacological approach to the genesis of ulcer disease II. A model study of stress-induced injury to gastric mucosa in rats." *Ann of the NY Acad of Scis*, 1990, 597:264-81.

[120] Tremblay A; et al."Regulation of rat adrenal messenger RNA and protein levels for cytochrome P-450s and adrenodoxin by dietary sodium depletion or potassium intake." *Jnl of Biol Chem*, 1991 Feb 5, 266(4):2245-51.

[121] Ziment I."History of the treatment of chronic bronchitis." *Respiration*, 1991, 58 Sup 1:37-42.

[122] Schwartz J; Weiss ST."Dietary factors and their relation to respiratory symptoms. The 2nd National Health and Nutr Examination Survey." *Amer Jnl of Epidemiology*, 1990 Jul, 132):67-76.

[123] Condron RJ."X-ray microanalytical Invest of the response of chicken proximal tubule cells to infection with avian infectious bronchitis virus." *Jnl of Submicroscopic Cyt and Path*, 1991 Jan, 23(1):159-65.

[124] Bertoni JM; Sprenkle PM."Low level lead inhibits the Hum brain cation pump." *Life Scis*, 1991, 48(22):2149.

[125] Personal interviews with Jim Lake and Hans Nieper, April 1992.

[126] Capurro C; Dorr R; Parisi M."Increased glucose transfer in the rat jejunum after dietary potassium loading: effect of amiloride." *Biochimica et Biophysica Acta*, 1991 May 31, 1065(1):1.

[127] Rajeswari P et al."Glucose induces lipid peroxidation and inactivation of Memb-associated ion-transport enzymes in Hum erythrocytes in vivo and in vitro." *Jnl of Cellular Phys*, 1991 Oct, 149(1):100-9.

[128] Adeeb N et al."Effect of age, weight, race and sex on blood pressure and erythrocytesodium pump characteristics." *Clin and Exper Hypert. Part A, Theory and Practice*, 1990,12(6):1115-34.

[129] Weinsier RL; et al. "Obesity-related Hypert: evaluation of the separate effects of energy restriction and weight reduction on hemodynamic and neuroendocrine status." *Amer Jnl of Med*, 1991 Apr, 90(4):460-8.

[130] Wassertheil-Smoller S; et al."Effect of antihypertensives on sexual function and quality of life: the TAIM Study." *Ann of Int Med*, 1991 Apr 15, 114(8):613-20.

[131] Norbiato G et al. "Effects of potassium Supation on insulin binding and insulin action in Hum obesity." *Eur Jnl of Clin Invest*, 1984, 44:414-9.

[132] Pasquali R; et al. "Erythrocyte Na+,K+-ATPase Memb activity in obese patients fed over a long term period with a very low caloric diet." *Metabolism*, 1988, 37:86-90.

[133] Waki M; et al."Relative expansion of extracellular fluid in obese vs. nonobese women." *Amer Jnl of Phys*, 1991 Aug, 261(2 Pt 1):E199.

[134] Kotchen TA; Kotchen JM; Boegehold MA."Nutr and Hypert Prev." *Hypert*, 1991 Sep, 18(3 Sup):I115-20.

[135] Sheehy TW. "Alcohol and the heart: How it helps, how it harms." *Postgr Med*, 1992 Apr, 91(5):271-77.

[136] Ettinger PO et al. "Arrhythmias and the 'Holiday Heart': alcohol-associated cardiac rhythm disorders." *Amer Heart Jnl*, 1978, 95(5):555-62.

[137] Gettes LS."Electrolyte abnormalities underlying lethal and ventricular arrhythmias." *Circ*, 1992 Jan, 85(1 Sup):I70-6.

[138] Komaru T et al."Role of ATP-sensitive potassium channels in coronary microvascular autoregulatory responses. *Circ Res*, 1991 Oct, 69(4):1146-51.

[139] Curtis MJ."The rabbit dual coronary perfusion model: a new method for assessing the pathological relevance of individual products of the ischaemic milieu: role of potassium in arrhythmogenesis.
" *Cardiov Res*, 1991 Dec, 25(12):1010-22.

[140] Grant AO Jr."On the mechanism of action of antiarrhythmic agents." *Amer Heart Jnl*, 1992 Apr, 123(4 Pt 2):1130-6.

[141] Busch AE; Ullrich F; Mutschler E."Antiarrhythmic properties of triamterene derivatives in the coronary artery ligated rat model." *Archiv der Pharmazie*, 1991 Nov, 324(11):895-8.

[142] Sanguinetti MC."Modulation of potassium channels by antiarrhythmic and antihypertensive drugs.*Hypert*, 1992 Mar, 19(3):228-36.

[143] Lamminpaa A; Vilska J."Acid-base balance in alcohol users seen in an emergency room." *Vet and Hum Tox*, 1991 Oct, 33(5):482-5.

[144] Bahr M et al."Central pontine myelinolysis associated with low potassium levels in alcoholism." *Jnl of Neurology*, 1990 Jul, 237(4):275-6.

[145] Ragland G."Electrolyte abnormalities in the alcoholic patient.
Emergency Med Clin of North America, 1990 Nov, 8(4):761-73.

[146] Laso FJ et al."Inter-relationship between serum potassium and plasma catecholamines and 3':5' cyclic monophosphate in alcohol withdrawal." *Drug and Alcohol Dependence*, 1990 Oct, 26(2):183-8.

[147] Roussaux JP; Derely M; Hers D.["Potassium chlorazepate administered orally in alcoholic detoxification"].
Jnl de Pharmacie de Belgique, 1989 May-Jun, 44(3):192-6.

[148] Nordrehaug J et al. "Serum potassium concentration as a risk factor of ventricular arrhythmias early in acute myocardial infarction." *Circ*, 1985, 71(4):645-9.

[149] Chen L.["Early effects of explosion on hearing threshold and activities of Na+-K+-ATPase and succinic dehydrogenase in the stria vascularis of guinea pigs."]Chung Hua Erh Pi Yen Hou Ko Tsa Chih *Chinese Jnl of Otorhinolaryngology*, 1991, 26(2):70-2, 124.

[150] Tungland OP; Savage MO; Bellman SC."A new syndrome: hearing loss and familial salivary gland insensitivity to aldosterone in two brothers." *Jnl of Laryngology and Otology*, 1990 Dec, 104:956-8.

[151] Yanick P. "Holistic applications to ear disorders. *Jnl of the Inter Acad of Prev Med*, 1983, 24.

[152] Lefebvre PP et al."Potassium-induced release of an endogenous toxic activity for outer hair cells and auditory neurons in the cochlea: a new pathoPhysl mechanism.in Meniere's disease?" *Hearing Res*, 1990 Aug 1, 47(1-2):83-93.

[153] Mark HE."Inner ear as an electrosensory sense organ." *Laryngo- Rhino- Otologie*, 1991 Jul, 70:340-9.

[154] WMCA, NY interview with William Oliver, M.D., on the Nutr 57, Betty Kamen Show.

[155] Jansson B. "Dietary, total body, and intracellular potassium-to-sodium ratios and their influence on Canc." *Canc Detection and Prev*, 1990, 14(5):563-5.

[156] Ariyoshi Y."Metabolic disturbance as paraneoplastic syndrome."*Jap Jnl of Canc and ChemoTher*, 1991 Mar, 18(3):350-6.

[157] Goncalves EL et al."Body composition in various Nutral conditions. Exper study."*Revista Paulista de Medicina*, 1990 May-Jun, 108(3):125-33.

[158] Pancrazio JJ et al."Voltage-dependent ion channels in small-cell lung Canc cells." *Canc Res*, 1989 Nov 1, 49:5901-6.

[159] Coggon D et al."Stomach Canc and food storage. " *Jnl of the National Canc Institute*, 1989 Aug 2, 81(15):1178-82.

[160] Kune GA; Kune S; Watson LF."Dietary sodium and potassium intake and colorectal Canc risk." *Nutr and Canc*, 1989, 12(4):351-9.

[161] Wrenn KD et al."The ability of Phys to predict electrolyte deficiency from the ECG"*Ann of Emergency Med*, 1990 May, 19:580-3.

[162] Usatiuk OV; Tsvilikhovskii NI; Melnichuk DA [The age-related characteristics of the transport ATPase activity in the enterocyte plasma Membs of the small intestine].*Biulleten Eksperimentalnoi Biologii i Meditsiny*, 1991 Mar, 111(3):309-11.

[163] Kamen B; Kamen S. *Kids Are What They Eat: What Every Parent Needs to Know About Nutr* (NY: Arco, 1983).

[164] Lucio FJ; Hendry BM; Ellory JC."The effects of cholesterol depletion on the sodium pump in human red cells." *Exper Phys*, 1991 May, 76(3):437.

[165] Tobian L et al."High K diets markedly reduce atherosclerotic cholesterol ester depositionin aortas of rats with hypercholest- erolemia and Hypert." *Amer Jnl of Hypert*, 1990 Feb, 3(2):133.

[166] Tobian L; Jahner TM; Johnson MA."Atherosclerotic cholesterol ester deposition is markedly reduced with a high-potassium diet. " *Jnl of Hypert*. Sup, 1989 Dec, 7(6):S244-5.

[167] Moskowitz MA."Basic mechanisms in vascular headache. " *Neur Clin*, 1990 Nov, 8(4):801-15.

[168] Leathard HL."New possibilities for anti-migraine drugs: prostanoid antagonists and progester-one-mimicking stabilizers of excitable cells." *Drug Design and Delivery*, 1989 Mar, 4(2):85-91.

[169] Luft FC. "Sodium, Chloride, and Potassium," in *Present Knowledge in Nutr*, 6th ed [[[etc.

[170] Morimoto S; Ogihara T.["Physl and pathological aging and electrolyte metabolism."]*Nippon Ronen Igakkai Zasshi*. Jap Jnl of Gers, 1991 May, 28(3):325-30.

[171] Krishna G et al. "Potassium Depletion Exacerbates Essential Hypert." *Ann of Int Med*, 1991 Jul, 115(2):77.

[172] Macquart-Moulin G et al. "Colorectal polyps and diet: a case-control study in Marseilles." *Inter Jnl of Canc*, 1987 Aug 15, 40(2):179-88.

[173] Caffery BE. "Influence of diet on tear function. " *Optometry and Vision Sci*, 1991 Jan, 68(1):58.

[174] Ibid.

[175] Kasuya M et al. "Changes of glutathione and taurine concentrations in lenses of rat eyes induced by galactose-cataract formation or ageing. " *Exper Eye Res*, 1992 Jan, 54(1):49-53.

[176] Kotler DP et al. "Preservation of short-term energy balance in Clinly stable patients with AIDS. " *AJCN*, 1990 Jan, 51(1):7-13.

[177] Guerra I; Kimmel PL. "Hypokalemic adrenal crisis in a patient with AIDS. " *S Med Jnl*, 1991 Oct, 84(10):1265-7.

[178] Cousens, G. *Conscious Eating* (Santa Rosa, CA: Vision Books Inter, 1992), p 119.

[179] Bech K et al. ["The pH and acidity of feces in colorectal neoplasms."] *Ugeskrift for Laeger*, 1990 Jan 15, 152:161-2.

[180] Lamminpaa A; Vilska J. "Acid-base balance in alcohol users seen in an emergency room." *Vet and Hum Tox*, 1991 Oct, 33(5):482-5.

[181] Redondo-Muller C et al. "In vitro maturation of the potential for movement of carp spermatozoa." *Mol Repro and Devel*, 1991 Jul, 29(3):259-70.

[182] Bringer J; et al. ["Influence of abnormal weight and imbalanced diet on female fertility."] *Presse Mede*, 1990 Sep 29, 19):1456-9.

[183] Stewart DE et al. "Infertility and eating disorders." *Amer Jnl of Obstetrics and Gynecology*, 1990 Oct, 163(4 Pt1):1196-9.

[184] Swanson LV. "Interactions of Nutr and Repro. *Jnl of Dairy Sci*, 1989 Mar, 72(3):805-14.

[185] Kalla NR; Dingley P; Ranga A. "Effect of gossypol on rats maintained on protein deficient and low potassium diets. " *Jnl of Dairy Sci*, 1989, *Acta Europaea Fertilitatis*, 1990 Mar-Apr, 21:85-9.

[186] Kaur S. "Effect of gossypol on the concentration of sodium and potassium in the rat epididymis. " *Inter Jnl of Andrology*, 1989 Aug, 12(4):318-20.

[187] McGarvey ST; et al. "Maternal prenatal dietary potassium, calcium, magnesium, and infant blood pressure. " *Hypert*, 1991 Feb, 17(2):218-24.

[188] Nicholas KR. "Milk secretion in the rat: progressive changes in milk composition during lactation and weaning and the effect of diet. " *Comp BioChem and Phys. a: Comp Phys*, 1991,98(3-4):535-42.

[189] Flyvbjerg A; et al. "Evidence that potassium deficiency induces growth retardation through reduced circulating levels of growth hormone and insulin-like growth factor I." *Metabolism: Clin and Exper*, 1991 Aug, 40(8):769-75.

[190] Mazzanti L; et al. "Sodium metabolism in offspring of hypertensive parents." *Bio Med and Metabolic Biol*, 1991 Apr, 45(2):181-7.

[191] Pennington JA; Young BE; Wilson DB. "Nutral elements in U.S. diets: results from the Total Diet Study,1982 to 1986. " *Jnl of the Amer Dietetic Assoc*, 1989 May, 89(5):659-64.

[192] Patterson TL; et al. "Aggregation of dietary calories, fats, and sodium in Mexican-Amer and Anglo families." *Amer Jnl of Prev Med*, 1988 Mar-Apr, 4(2):75-82.

[193] Moses N; Banilivy M; Lifshitz F. "Fear of obesity among adolescent girls." *Pediatrics*, 1989, 83:393-8.

[194] Maloney M; et al. "Dieting behavior and eating attitudes in children." *Pediatrics*, 1989, 84:482.

[195] Pugliese M; et al. "Fear of obesity: a cause of short stature and delayed puberty." *NEJM*, 1983, 309:513-18.

[196] Patrick J; Golden MHV. "Leukocyte electrolytes and sodium transport in protein energy malnutr." *AJCN*, 1977, 30:1478-81.

[197] Gomez-Marin O et al. "The Sodium-Potassium Bld Pres Trial in Children. Design, recruitment, and randomization: The children and adolescent blood pressure program. " *Controlled Clin Trials*, 1991 Jun, 12(3):408-23.

[198] Lifshitz F et al. "Nutral dwarfing: a growth abnormality associated with reduced erythrocyte Na+, K+-ATPase activity[1-3]." *AJCN*, 1991, 54:997-1004.

PART III

[1] Warwick PM. "Dietary intake of individuals interested in eating a healthy diet: a validated study of intake before and after dietary advice." *Hum Nutr. Applied Nutr*, 1987 Dec, 41:409-25.

[2] Pichard C; et al. "Intracellular potassium and Memb potential in rat muscles during malNutr and subsequent refeeding." *AJCN*, 1991 Sep, 54(3):489-98.

[3] "Salt and Hypert." *Nutr Action*, Apr 1981, 8:3-4.

[4] Levine AS; Labuza TP."Food systems: the relationship between health and food Sci/technology." *Envir Health Perspectives*, 1990 Jun, 86:233-8.

[5] Rusul G; Marth EH."Food additives and plant components control growth and aflatoxin production by toxigenic aspergilli: a Rev.*Mycopathologia*, 1988 Jan, 101(1):13-23.

[6] Eaton SB; Shostak M; Konner M. *The Paleolithic Prescription: A Program of Diet & Exercise and a Design for Living* (NY: Harper & Row, Publ, 1988), p 81.

[7] "Gourmet Foods Now TV Dinners," *Wall Street Jnl*, May 5, 1967

[8] Witschi JC et al. "Sources of sodium, potassium, and energy in the diets of adolescents." *Jnl of the Amer Dietetic Assoc*, 1987 Dec, 87(12):1651-5.

[9] Jollife; Tisdall; Cannon. *Clin Nutr* (NY: Paul Hober Books), p 127.

[10] National Res Council, "Recommended Dietary Allowances," 10th ed, National Acad Press, Wash, D.C., 1989.

[11] Debry G.["Nutral requirements of aged people"].*Neph*, 1990, 11(5):307-11.

[12] Moore R; Webb G. *The K Factor* (NY: Macmillan, 1986), p 215.

[13] Scala J. *High Blood Pressure Relief Diet* (NY: Penguin, 1990), p 52.

[14] Halpern SL. *Quick Reference to Clin Nutr: A Guide for Phys* (Phil: JB Lippencott Co, 1979).

[15] Scala J. *High Bld Press Relief Diet* (NY: Penguin, 1990), p 51.

[16] Jansson B. "Dietary, total body, and intracellular potassium-to-sodium ratios and their influence on Canc." *Canc Detection and Prev*, 1990, 14(5):563-5.

[17] Inter Commission on Radiation Protection (1975). Report of the Task Force Group on Reference Man, no 23, Pergamon Press, Oxford.

[18] Meneely G; Battarbee H. "Sodium and potassium." *Nutr Revs, 1976*, 34:225-35.

[19] *Present Knowledge in Nutr*, ed Brown ML. Inter Life Scis Institute, Nutr Foundation, Wash, D.C. (1990):442.

[20] Harvey RA; Theuer RC."Potassium as an index of fruit content in baby food products. Part I.Banana-containing and apricot-containing products." *Jnl Assoc of Official Analytical Chemists*, 1991 Nov-Dec,74(6):929.

[21] Robson JRK. *MalNutr: Its Causation and Control* (NY: Gordon and Breach, 1972), p 528.

[22] Sangiori GB et al. "Serum potassium levels, red-blood-cell potassium and alterations of the repolarization phase of electrocardiography in old subjects." *Age Aging*, 1984, 13:309.

[23] Fellers PJ; Nikdel S; Lee HS."Nutrient content and Nutr labeling of several processed Florida citrus juice products." *Jnl of the Amer Dietetic Assoc*, 1990 Aug, 90(8):1079-84.

[24] Hunter, BT. *Consumer Beware* (NY: Simon & Schuster, 1971), p 276.

[25] Vertut-Doi A; Hannaert P; Bolard J."The polyene antibiotic amphotericin B inhibits the Na+/K+ pump of human erythrocytes." *Bio and BioPhys Res Communications*, 1988 Dec 15, 157(2):692.

[26] Ginter E.["Nutr in the Prev of ischemic heart disease."]*Bratislavske Lekarske Listy*, 1989 Mar, 90(3):203-21.

[27] Quillin P. *Healing Nutrients*. (NY: Random House, 1989), p 73.

[28] Kimura M; Itokawa Y."Cooking losses of mins in foods and its Nutral significance." *Jnl of Nutral Sci and Vitaminology*, 1990, 36 Sup 1:S25-32;discussion S33.

[29] Ahern DA; Kaley LA. "Electrolyte content of salt-replacement seasonings." *Jnl of the Amer Dietetic Assoc*, 1989 Jul, 89:935-8.

[30] Scala J. *High Bld Pressure Relief Diet* (NY: Penguin, 1990), p 87.

[31] Halpern SL. *Quick Reference to Clin Nutr: A Guide for Phys* (Phil: JB Lippencott Co., 1979).

[32] Abdulla M; Behbehani A; Dashti H."Dietary intake and bioavailability of trace elements." *Biol Trace Element Res*, 1989 Jul-Sep, 21:173.

[33] Pak CY."Citrate and renal calculi: new insights and future directions." *Amer Jnl of Kidney Diseases*, 1991 Apr, 17(4):420-5.

[34] Lemann J Jr et al."Potassium bicarbonate, but not sodium bicarbonate, reduces urinary calcium excretion and improves calcium balance in healthy men." *Kidney Inter*, 1989 Feb, 35:688-95.

[35] *Nutr Revs*, "Present Knowledge in Nutr," 5th ed, The Nutr Foundation, Inc., Wash, D.C., 1984. Reynolds, J, ed, "Martindale: The Extra Pharmacopeia," 29th ed, The Pharm Press, London, 1989.

[36] Menon M; Mahle CJ. "Urinary citrate excretion in patients with renal calculi." *Jnl of Urology*, 1983, 129(6):1158-60.

[37] Roe DA. *Drug Induced Nutral Deficiencies* (Westpt, Conn: The Avi Publ Co, Inc, 1978), p 17.

[38] Krotkiewski M; et al."Effects of a sodium-potassium ion-exchanging seaweed preparation in mild Hypert." *Amer Jnl of Hypert*, 1991 Jun, 4(6):483-8.

[39] Liebermeister H[Cardiac effects of a reducing diet].*Versicherungsmedizin*, 1991 Jun 1, 43(3):71.

[40] Pak CY et al."Effect of meal on the Physl and physicochem actions of potassium citrate." *Jnl of Urology*, 1991 Sep, 146:803-5.

[41] Krause Mv; Mahan LK. *Food, Nutr and Diet Ther* (Phil: WB Saunders Co, 19 79) p 123.

[42] Rude RK."Phys of magnesium metabolism and the important role of magnesium in potassium deficiency." *Amer Jnl of Card*, 1989 Apr 18, 63(14):31G-34G.

[43] Pennington JA. *Dietary Nutrient Guide* (Westpt, Conn: The Avi Publ Co, Inc, 1976), p 50.

[44] Dychner T; Wester PO. "Magnesium and potassium in serum and muscle in relation to disturbances of cardiac rhythm." In *Magnesium in Health and Disease* (Shils, Maine: *Spectrum Publ Co*, 1980), 551-7.

[45] Wester PO. "Intracellular electrolytes in cardiac failure."*Acta Medica Scan*, 1986, 707:33-36.

[46] Pennington JA. Op cit.

[47] Kumanyika S."Behavioral aspects of intervention strategies to reduce dietary sodium."*Hypert*, 1991 Jan, 17(1 Sup):I190-5.

[48] Hegsted DM."A perspective on reducing salt intake." *Hypert*, 1991 Jan, 17(1 Sup):I201-4.

[49] Haddy FJ. "Roles of sodium, potassium, calcium, and natriuretic factors in Hypert." *Hypert*, 1991 Nov, 18(5 Sup):III179-83.

[50] Siani A; et al."Increasing the dietary potassium intake reduces the need for antihypertensive medication." *Ann of Int Med*, 1991 Nov 15, 115(10):753-9.

[51] Pak CY et al."Effect of meal on the Physl and physicochemical actions of potassium citrate." *Jnl of Urol*, 1991 Sep, 146:803-5.

[52] McCarron DA. "The integrated effects of electrolytes on blood pressure." *The Nutr Report*, 1991 Aug, 9(8):57,62,64.

[53] Blake GH; Beebe DK. "Management of Hypert. Useful nonpharmacologic measures." *Postgr Med*, 1991 Jul, 90(1):151-4, 158.

[54] Liebermeister H; Bleckmann A.["Cardiac effects of a reducing diet"].*Versicherungsmedizin*, 1991 Jun 1, 43(3):71-5.

[55] Cappuccio FP; MacGregor GA. "Does potassium Supation lower blood pressure? A meta-analysis of published trials." *Jnl of Hypert*, 1991 May, 9(5):465-73.

[56] Lowik MR; et al."Nutr and blood pressure among elderly men and women" (Dutch NutrSurveillance System).*Jnl of the Amer Col of Nutr*, 1991 Apr, 10(2):149-55.

[57] Valdes G; et al. "Potassium Supation lowers blood pressure and increases urinary kallikrein in essential hypertensives." *Jnl of Hum Hypert*, 1991 Apr, 5(2):91-6.

[58] Obel AO; Koech DK. "Potassium Supation versus bendrofluazide in mildly to moderately hypertensive Kenyans." *Jnl of Cardiov Pharm*, 1991 Mar, 17(3):504 7.

[59] Shah J; Jandhyala BS."Role of Na+,K(+)-ATPase in the centrally mediated hypotensive effects of potassium in anaesthetized rats." *Jnl of Hypert*, 1991 Feb, 9(2):167-70.

[60] Sato Y; et al."High-potassium diet attenuates salt-induced acceleration of Hypert in SHR." *Amer Jnl of Phys*, 1991 Jan, 260(1 Pt 2):R21-6.

[61] Jacobs MM."Potassium inhibition of DMH-induced small intestinal tumors in rats."*Nutr and Canc*, 1990, 14(2):95-101.

[62] Heseltine F. "Potassium Supation in the treatment of idiopathic postural hypotension."*Age and Aging*, 1990, 19:409-14.

[63] Cheng HM; Jap TS; Ho LT. "Fanconi syndrome: report of a case." *Taiwan i Hsueh Hui Tsa Chih Jnl of the Formosan Med Assoc*, 1990 Dec, 89(12):1115-7.

[64] Greminger P; et al. ["Nutr and Hypert: what are the goals?"].*Schweizerische Rundschau fur Medizin Praxis*, 1990 Sep 11, 79:1055.

[65] O'Byrne S; Feely J."Effects of drugs on glucose tolerance in non-insulin-dependent diabetics(Part I)." *Drugs*, 1990 Jul, 40(1):6-18.

[66] Junker L; et al.["Serum enzymes in grade I hypertensive patients before and following a change in Nutr in relation to polyene acid and electrolyte content"].*Zeitschrift fur die Gesamte Innere Medizin und Ihre Grenzgebiete*, 1990 Jun 15, 45(11):323-4.

[67] Packer M."Potential role of potassium as a determinant of morbidity and mortality in patients with systemic Hypert and congestive heart failure." *Amer Jnl of Card*, 1990 Mar 6, 65(10):45E-51E; discussion 52E.

[68] Linas SL."Potassium: weighing the evidence for Supation." *Hospital Practice*, 1988 Dec 15, 23:73, 83-4, 86.

[69] Packer M."Potential role of potassium as a determinant of morbidity and mortality in patients with systemic Hypert and congestive heart failure." *Amer Jnl of Card*, 1990 Mar 6, 65(10):45E-51E; discussion 52E.

[70] Kies C; Harms JM."Copper absorption as affected by Supal calcium, magnesium, manganese, selenium and potassium." *Advances in Exper Med and Biol*, 1989, 258:45-58.

[71] Lemann J Jr et al."Potassium bicarbonate, but not sodium bicarbonate, reduces urinary calcium excretion and improves calcium balance in healthy men." *Kidney Inter*, 1989 Feb, 35:688-95.

[72] Linas SL."Potassium: weighing the evidence for Supation." *Hosp Prac* (Office Edition), 1988 Dec 15, 23(12):73-9, 83-4, 86.

[73] Eaton SB; Shostak M; Konner M. *The Paleolithic Prescription: A Program of Diet & Exercise and a Design for Living* (NY: Harper & Row, Publ, 1988), p 117.

[74] Harvey JA et al. "Calcium citrate: Reduced propensity for the crystallization of calcium oxalate in urine resulting from induced hypercalciuria of calcium Supation." *Jnl of Endoc Metabolism*, 1985, 61(6):1223-25.

[75] Tobian L et al. *"Potassium reduces cerebral hemorrhage and death rate in hypertensive rats, even when blood pressure is not lowered."* Hypert, 1985, 7(Sup I):I110—114.

[76] Preminger GM et al. *"Prev of recurrent calcium stone formation with potassium citrate Ther in patients with renal tubular acidosis."* Jnl of Urology, 1985, 134(1):20-23.

[77] Pac CYC; Fuller C. "Idiopathic hypocitraturic calcium-oxalate nephrolithiasis successfully treated with potassium citrate." *Ann of Int Med*, 1986, 104:33-37.

[78] Norbiato G et al. "Effects of potassium Supation on insulin binding and insulin action in Hum obesity." *Eur Jnl of Clin Invest*, 1984, 44:414-9.

[79] Khaw KT; Thom S. "Randomized double-blind cross-over trial of potassium on blood pressure in normal subjects." *Lancet*, 1982, 2:1127-29.

[80] Stoff JA. *Chronic Fatigue Syndrome: The Hidden Epidemic* (NY: Random House, 1988), p 114.

[81] Maxwell MH; Kleeman CR; Narins RG. *Clin Disorders of Fluid and Electrolyte Metabolism*, 1987, McGraw-Hill Book Co, NY.

[82] Moore RD; Webb GD. *The K Factor* (NY: Pocket Books, Simon & Schuster, 1986), p 365.

[83] Luft FC; McCarron DA."Heterogeneity of Hypert: the diverse role of electrolyte intake." *Annual Rev of Med*, 1991, 42:347-55.

[84] Mazzanti L; et al. "Effect of magnesium-deficient diet on cation transport in pregnant rabbits." *Magnesium Res*, 1991 Mar, 4(1):45.

[85] Sullivan PA et al."Strenuous short-term dynamic exercise: effects on heart rate, blood pressure, potassium homeostasis, and packed cell volume in mild Hypert." *Jnl of Hypert*. Sup, 1989 Dec, 7(6):S90-1.

[86] Makarovskii VV et al.["Dynamics of hormones, sugar and electrolytes during hypodynamia according to blood Bio indices"].*Kosmicheskaia Biologiia i Aviakosmicheskaia Meditsina*, 1987 Jan-Feb, 21(1):21-7.

[87] Miric M; Haxhiu MA.["Effect of vitamin C on exercise-induced bronchoconstriction"].*Plucne Bolesti*, 1991 Jan-Jun, 43(1-2):94-7.

[88] Rugg-Gunn A. "Empty calories? Nutrient intake in relation to sugar intake in English adolescents." *Jnl of Hum Nutr and Dietetics*, 1991, 4:101-11.

[89] Ericsson Y et al."Urinary min ion loss after sugar ingestion." *Bone and Min*, 1990 Jun, 9(3):233.

[90] Rorsman F; Hellman B."Glucose-induced increase of potassium in pancreatic beta-cells associated with reduced mobilization of the ion." *BioChem Inter*, 1988 Jan, 16(1):93-9.

[91] Bordoni A et al. "Effect of a hyperlipidic diet on lipid composition, fluidity, and (Na+-K+)ATPase activity of rat erythrocyte Membs." *Memb BioChem*, 1989, 8(1):11-8.

[92] Nicholas KR; Hartmann PE."Milk secretion in the rat: progressive changes in milk composition during lactation and weaning and the effect of diet." *Comp BioChem and Phys. a: Comp Phys*, 1991,98(3-4):535-42.

[93] Zholos AV; Baidan LV; Shuba MF."The inhibitory action of caffeine on calcium currents in isolated intestinal smooth muscle cells." *Eur Jnl of Phys*, 1991 Oct, 419(3-4):267-73.

[94] Ishihara H; Karaki H."Inhibitory effect of 8-(N,N-diethylamino)octyl-3,4,5-trimethoxybenzoate (TMB-8) in vascular smooth muscle." *Eur Jnl of Pharm*, 1991 May 17, 197(2-3):181-6.

[95] Nussberger J."Caffeine-induced diuresis and atrial natriuretic peptides." *Jnl of Cardiov Pharm*, 1990 May, 15(5):685-91

[96] Yeh JK et al. *Jnl of Nutr*, 1986, 116(2):273-80.

Index